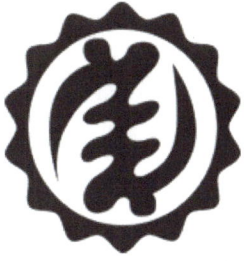

ANESTHESIA TECHNICIAN
SURVIVAL GUIDE

By Anesthesia Technicians for Anesthesia Technicians

ESAI GLOBAL LLC PUBLISHINGS

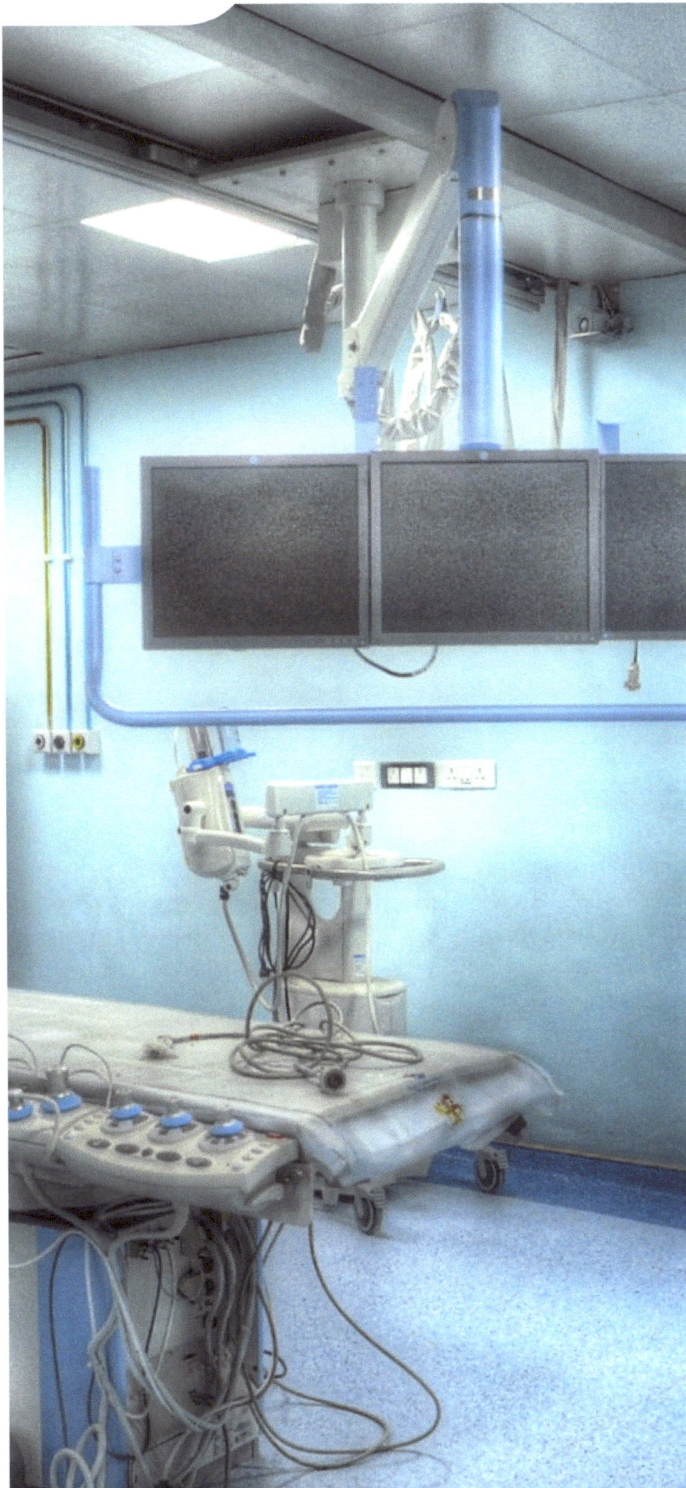

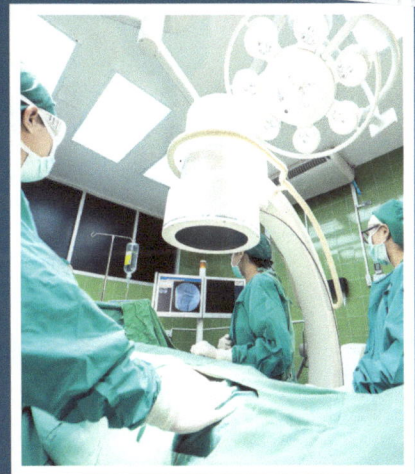

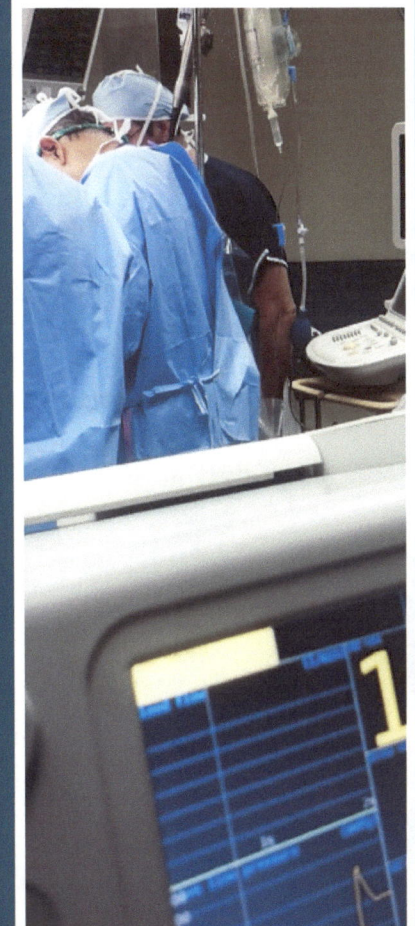

Third Edition

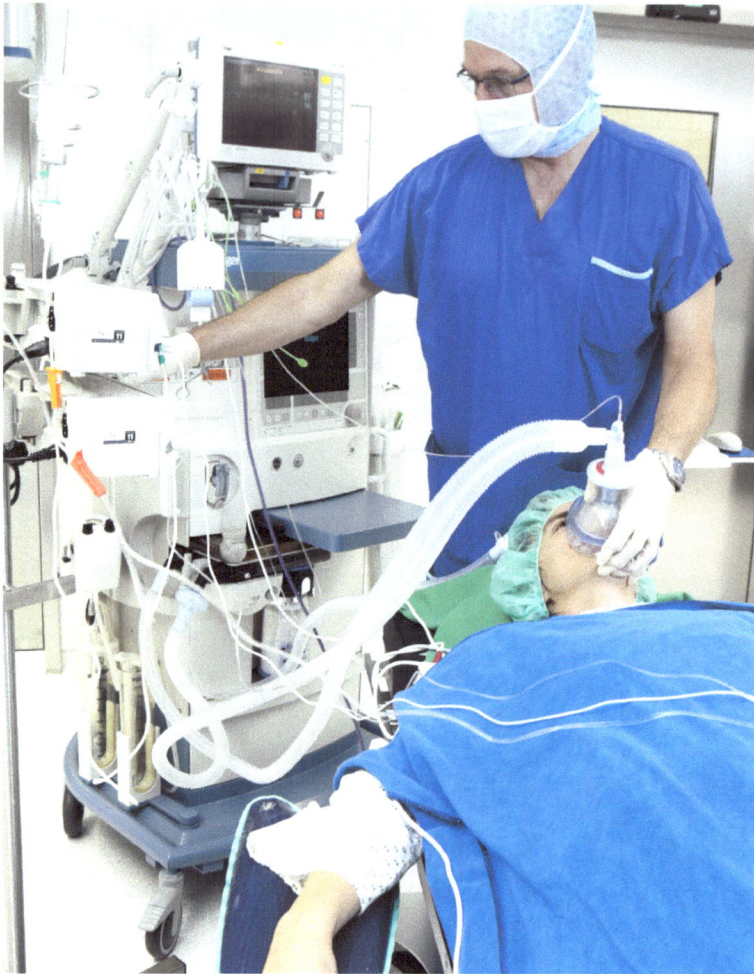

Editors

DR. JEREMY WILLIAMS

Professor North West Fitness Institute

KEMPHOR HASKINS

Anesthesia Technician

ALBERT PHAM

Anesthesia Technician

TORIN GAYLES

Anesthesia Technician

LANCE GRANGER

Anesthesia Technician

Anesthesia Technician Survival Guide Copyright © 2017 by Tony Pang

MESAI Global LLC Press

DEDICATION

Mama, this is for you. Thank you for constantly being there for me, and thank you for the bean pies.

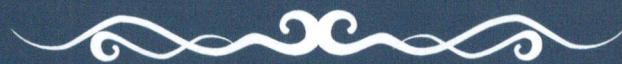

PREFACE

As the chief technician at Strong Memorial Hospital, one of my responsibilities was to supervise the preparation of all our anesthesia technicians. I saw there was a great deal of data to process and remember as an anesthesia tech. I also found that everyone was at different levels in their training. I said to myself, "I wish there was a smaller companion book to go along with our large anesthesia training manual to help our techs as they proceed in their training." Of course, there wasn't one, so I decided to write one, with the help of my good friend, RN Patrick Furbert. With the completion of that project, I went on to develop a smaller, less detailed anesthesia technician survival guide that anesthesia technicians all over the world can use.

The purpose of this anesthesia technician survival guide is to support the anesthesia technician as they continue their education and to help them better perform their duties in the operating room environment. This book is intended to be a guide and not to supersede their hospital individual training, policy, procedures or protocols

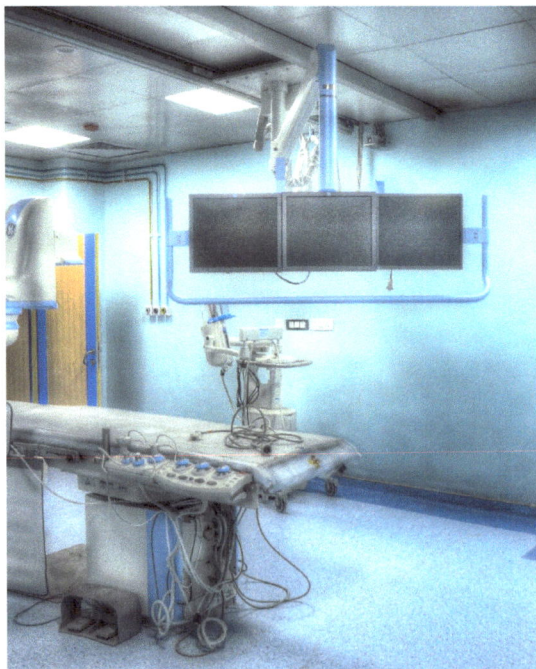

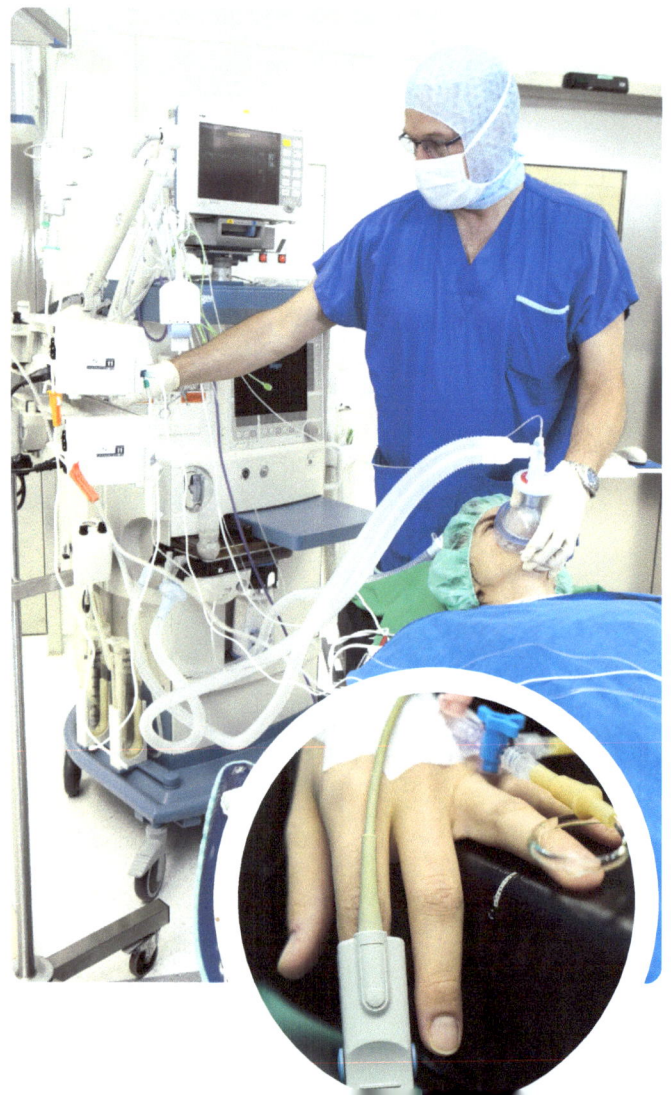

ACKNOWLEDGEMENTS

I would like to acknowledge the anesthesia department at the University of Rochester Medical Center for everything you have done for me. Thanks to Alicia Arrington and Chris Nations at Oakwood Hospital for all your patience and support. Thank you, Elsa Pang. I could not have done this without you. To Erskine Ford, my best friend and writing inspiration. A big thank you to Dr. Liz Elliot. Thank you a million, Ed Grin, my writing instructor and friend. Thank you, Meredith Egan, Katherine Aubrey, Bea Rhodes, Heartspeak Productions, Evelyn Zellers, Jane Miller, Simon Fraser, and the Center for Restorative Justice at Simon Fraser University.

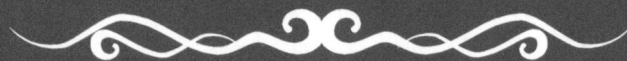

TABLE OF CONTENTS

TABLE OF CONTENTS

GENERAL TECHNICIAN DUTIES

Anesthesia technicians perform a variety of duties to assist other members of anesthesia care teams. Job duties might vary by an anesthesia technician's skill level, as well as the state and type of facility in which he or she is employed. In general, anesthesia technicians clean, sterilize, test, calibrate and troubleshoot anesthesia equipment, as well as keep records of equipment inspections. More advanced duties might include transporting patients to surgery, explaining procedures to patients and operating equipment, such as electronic and pneumatic devices that monitor patients who are under anesthesia.

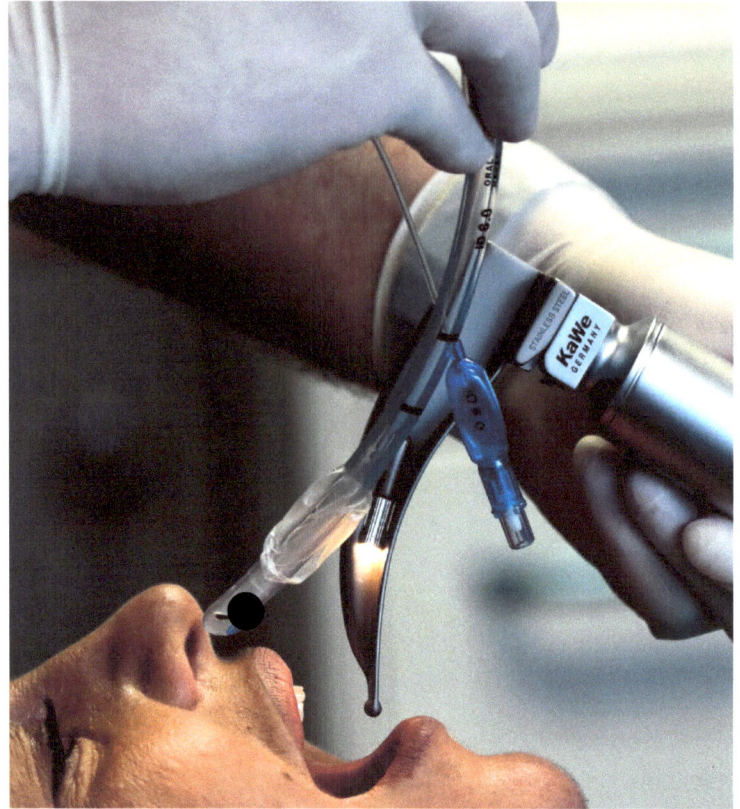

- Support the clinicians - priority
- Make sure your nameplate and your phone number are up and visible in every operating room you have been assigned.
- Verify network accessibility.
- Check the number of cases and type of cases.
- Turnover and re-stock anesthesia gas and anesthesia carts.
- Restock open or used airway boxes.
- Perform point of care testing (POCT) quality control tests.
- Restock OB anesthesia gas machines and anesthesia support carts, i.e., Pyxis, Omni, Block, A-line, and Airway carts
- Retrieve anesthesia equipment and supplies from common floors, Pre-Operative Care Unit (PRE-OP), Post-Anesthesia Care Unit (PACU)
- Verify availability of clean and working DCI scopes, glidescopes, laryngoscope handles, and blades (clinicians cannot intubate patients without clean handles and blades).
- Verify difficult intubation, and trauma carts stocked and in designated areas.
- Verify cell-saver, rapid infusers, and transducers are set up.
- Verify center cores have o2 tanks/retrieve viable tanks from PACU and SSC.
- Verify trauma rooms have required equipment.

01.

SHIFT DUTIES AND GOALS

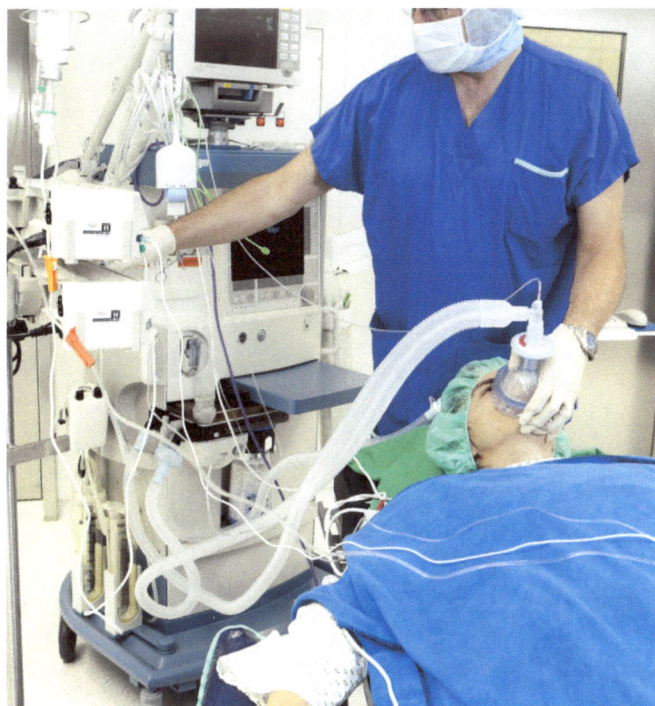

- Fill first case request (except Friday and Saturday overnight)
- Restock MRI cart
- Restock block cart
- Restock anesthesia supplies in the wall lockers in pre-anesthesia and PACU
- Refill arterial line totes
- Ectopic setup for the following day
- Close rooms the afternoons didn't get to
- Setup trauma and emergency rooms

02

Night Shift Specific Duties

- Check out anesthesia gas machines
- Support cases throughout the day
- Turnover rooms for cases to follow
- Refill arterial line totes
- Close rooms when possible
- Setup trauma and emergency rooms
- In the movie, it is Pearl who acts as the narrator of the story.

03.

Day Shift Specific Duties

- Support rooms that are still running
- Close rooms that are done for the day
- Refill arterial line totes
- Setup trauma and emergency rooms

POLICIES, PROCEDURES & PROTOCOLS

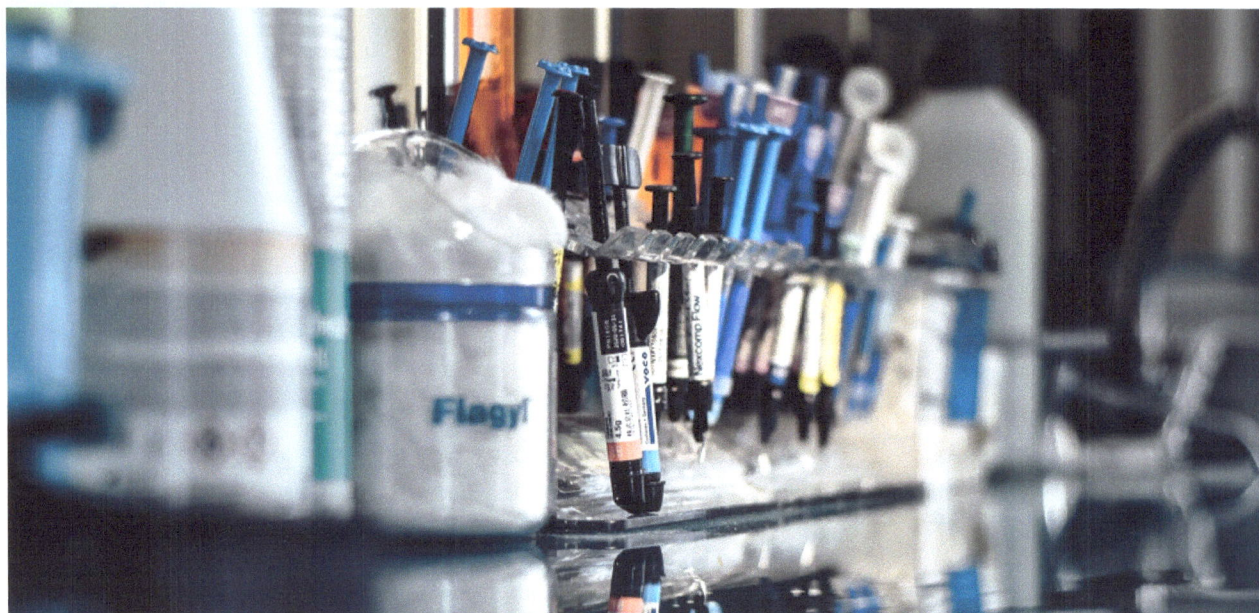

It is very important to learn your hospital policies, procedures and protocols as quickly as possible because learning these will greatly increase your overall learning of your job and what is expected of you. I have listed a few below that should be standard for any anesthesia technology department. Please refer to your department policies, procedures, and protocols.

HIPAA
Any information related to a patient's health CANNOT be used unless authorized by either the patient or someone acting on the patient's behalf, or unless permitted by regulation. (DO NOT DISCLOSE CONFIDENTIAL PATIENT INFORMATION.

OR Dress Code
Scrub tops with pants, hair con ned, no artificial fingernails, jewelry kept to a minimum. PPE (personal protective equipment) must be worn whenever there is a risk for exposure to patient blood or body fluid. Examples of PPE are gloves, face masks, eye shields, and gowns.

Code of Conduct
Employees are expected to work together to provide an environment free of inappropriate behavior, harassment, and discrimination. Disagreements should be handled with courtesy, respect, and dignity. Incidents of harassment or disruptive behavior must be reported to your supervisor immediately.

The Point of Care Testing

Blood gasses, ACTs, TEGs testing, and QC must be performed by certified anesthesia techs. The attending clinicians are the supervisors of the point of care testing.

Blood Cooler Delivery

Ensure the name of the patient on the blood cooler matches the name on the blood bags. If there is a mismatch, return cooler to the blood bank and notify them of the error. You MUST check to see if the name on the cooler matches the name of the patient in/entering the operating room. Ask a clinician for the patient's name (they must verify via the second identifier). Repeat the patient's MED-REC/patient ID number to the clinician for secondary verification.

Blood Gas Retrieval

Anesthesia technicians must verify blood gas syringes with a clinician with a second identifier before leaving the room. Refer to blood cooler delivery protocol. If there are any difficulties in carrying out this procedure, promptly report them to your supervisor.

Unsecured Controlled Drugs in OR

If a pack of unsecured controlled drugs (narcotics) is discovered, report it to the attending physician, clinical coordinator, and pharmacy tech immediately. Shift Change Over - Shift changeover will take place from 2:10 - 2:20 pm. 1st and 2nd shift techs must together go through each room in the core. Inspect rooms that have no more cases for missing or overstocked items.

Cell Phone Etiquette

When answering a call, you should say, "Anesthesia, this is YOUR NAME. How may I help you?"

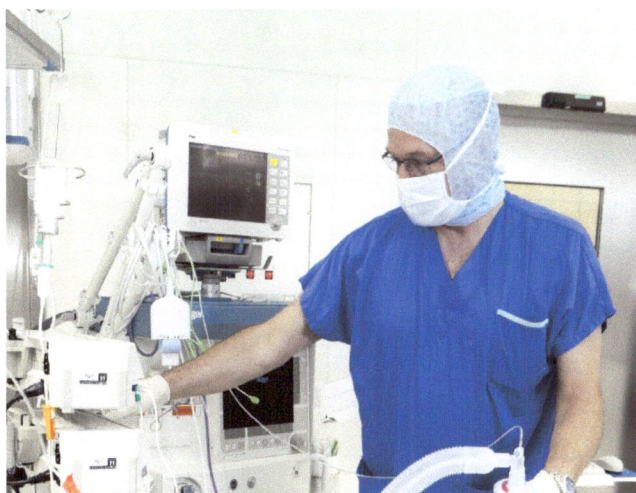

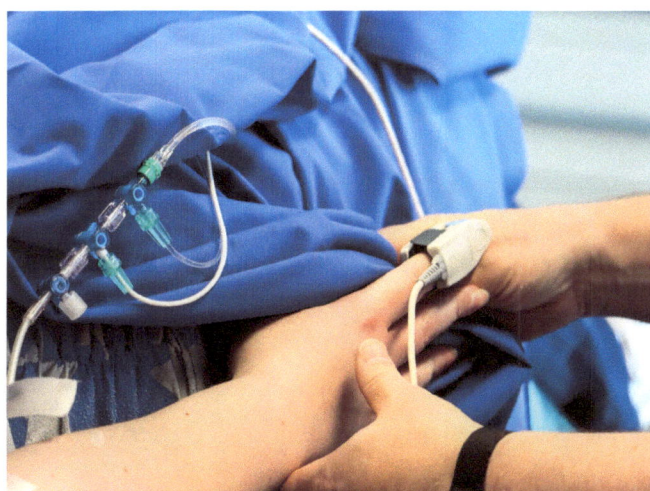

BASIC TRAINING

Cleaning Laryngoscope Handles and Blades

At the end of every case, soiled laryngoscope handles and blades must be retrieved and put in the dirty collection bin in the stock room. Handle covers must be separated from the battery packs. Techs responsible for cleaning the blades will take them to MPD (Material Processing Department) for processing. MPD personnel must be notified prior to the drop-o .

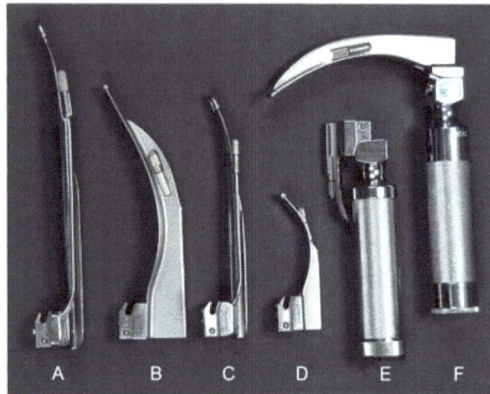

Glide and DCI Scope Maintenance

When transporting to MPD for processing, techs will need to place each soiled, labeled scope in its corresponding container with the lid secured. MPD personnel must be notified prior to delivery that scopes need to be processed. Finally, techs must witness MPD scan the barcode(s) corresponding to the appropriate scope(s) before leaving (if your hospital has a bar coding system.).

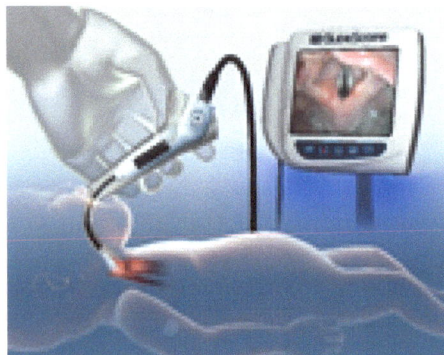

O2 Tanks

Each center core must be stocked with oxygen tanks. These tanks are supplied by Respiratory Care. If the supply of O2 tanks is empty, Respiratory Care must be paged and asked to deliver a new supply. Inform the tech of how many racks of tanks you need and where to bring them. Exchange empty racks for the full ones.

Equipment Tracking

Anesthesia equipment should be recorded on an equipment board or log. This includes anesthesia gas machines, Pyxis carts, glide scopes, blood gas analyzers, ACT machines, and glucometers.

Equipment Retrieval

Each shift is responsible for retrieving anesthesia equipment (transport monitors, defibrillators, Baxter/infusion pumps, transducer brackets, etc.). Grab a wire cart and head over to the equipment retrieval areas. For shift turnover, it is ideal to have a minimum of three monitors and defibrillators available. Whenever you are unable to nd equipment, search the other units on these floors.

Cart Stocking

Anesthesia carts; Pyxis, pediatric and block carts are labeled with stickers (usually orange) displaying item names and associated par level. Stock each labeled item to its appropriate par level.

Troubleshooting Common Anesthesia Gas Machine Problems

When it comes to troubleshooting the anesthesia gas machines, I have a few tips that I have learned over the years that are tried and tested that I stand by.

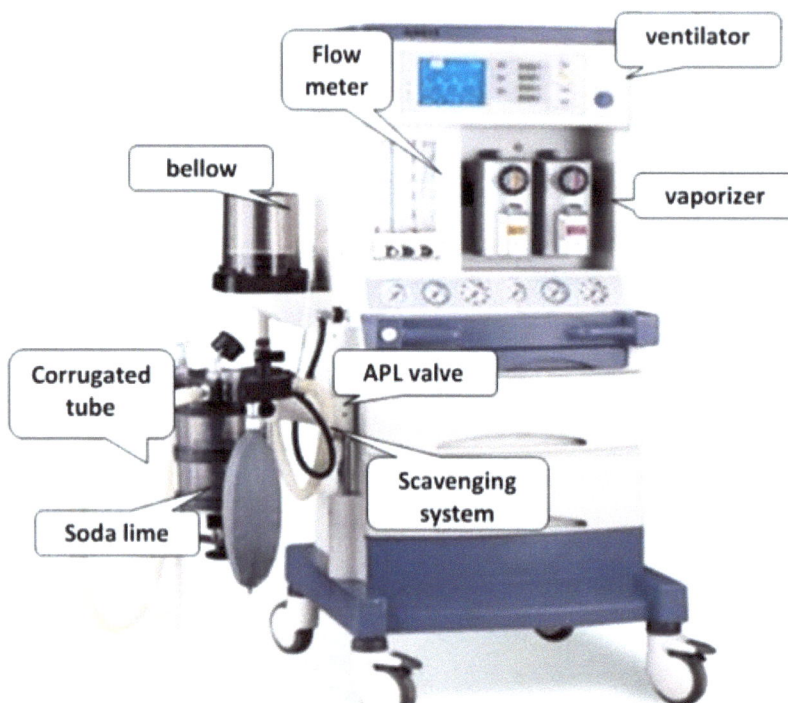

TIPS:

1) Daily cleaning will prevent 90 percent of all your problems, and a general deep cleaning at least once per month will greatly reduce errors and problems.

2) Whenever you have an error, start with the patient and work your way back to the machine.

3) If I get a call from a provider about an error or malfunction, I always bring replacement parts to the OR to save on time, and I take the damaged or broken parts to an empty OR to troubleshoot it there. Many providers appreciate that.

Low-Pressure Alarm

The low-pressure leak is the most common issue that I have come across in my experience with Aestiva, Aespire, ADU as well as Aisys anesthesia gas machines.

- Check for a low-pressure leak.
- Check the circuit (starting on the patient work your way back to the machine); make sure it is fully connected.
- Check the gas sample line.
- Check the bellows.
- Check the CO canister.
- Check flow sensors.
- Check oxygen pressure from pipeline and tank.
- Check ventilator relief.

VENTILATOR WON'T FILL

Most likely, there is a leak somewhere, so check for a low-pressure leak or check ventilator relief valve.

VENTILATOR WON'T DELIVER A BREATH

Most likely, there is too much moisture in circuit or flow valves or flow transducer. • Look for inspiratory reverse flow.
- Check for high airway pressure.
- Check for bad expiratory valve.
- Try changing the flow sensors.

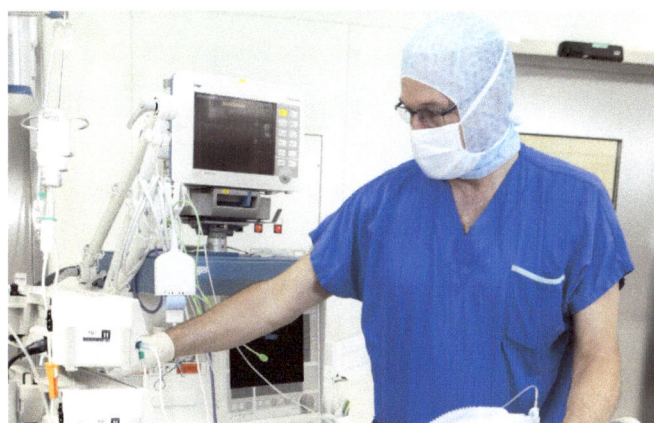

High Airway Pressure with Mechanical Ventilation

Most of the time, the cause of high airway pressure is patient related, and it is often resolved by the anesthesia provider and is not really in our scope of practice, but we can assist and check our equipment.

- Make sure the breathing circuit is not obstructed, bent, or kinked in any way.
- Glance at the ETT for obstructions, kinking, or secretions (if so inform the anesthesia provider; do not touch).
- Check pop-off valve.
- Check peep settings (PEEP = Positive End Expiratory Pressure).
- Check ventilator parameters.

High airway pressure

Triggered when resistance to ventilation is high

Causes

◦ **Ventilator problems:**

Inappropriate settings, excessive tidal volume, ventilator malfunction – rare

◦ **Circuit problems**

Fluid pooling in circuit/ filter,kinking of circuit

◦ **Endotracheal tube obstruction**

Due to sputum, kinking, biting

◦ **Increased airway resistance**

Bronchospasm, decreased respiratory system compliance, decreased chest wall compliance

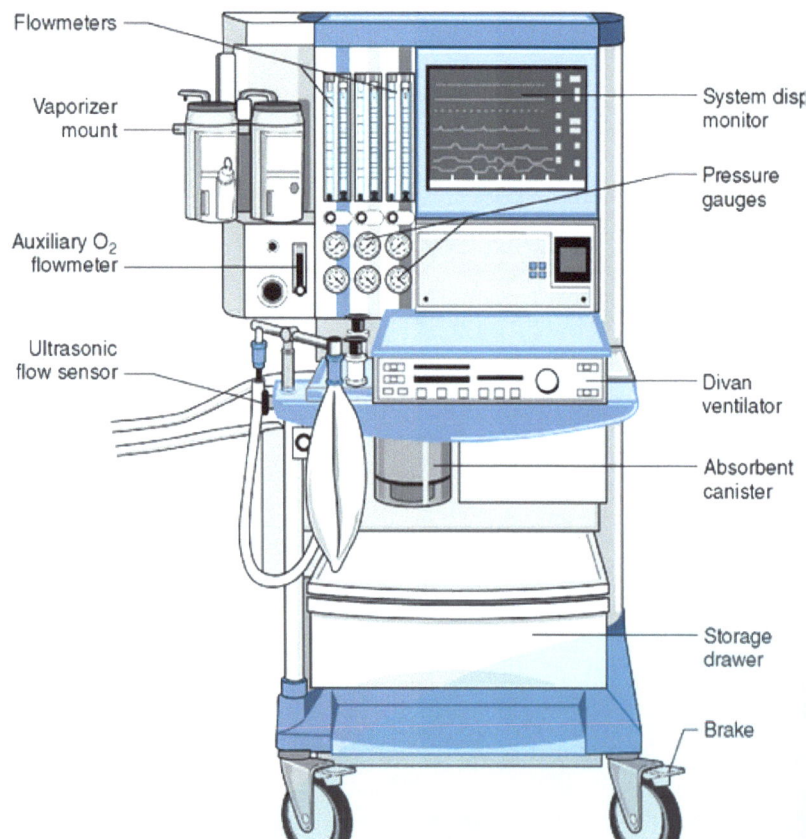

Flowmeter Problems

- Check for a leak.
- Check bobbin to see if it's stuck.

95% of the time, the float in the flow meter is stuck or clogged with debris. Tap the flow-meter a few times to see if you can free the float of debris. Some flowmeters can be easily replaced. If so, replace it and send the damaged one for cleaning and repairs.

Another cause could be a small crack in the flowmeter tube.

Flowmeters

Vaporizer mount

Auxiliary O_2 flowmeter

Ultrasonic flow sensor

System disp monitor

Pressure gauges

Divan ventilator

Absorbent canister

Storage drawer

Brake

Gas Analyzer Problems

No CO2 Tracing

The most common cause of problems with the gas analyzer I have found is moisture in the sample line

- Make sure the gas analyzer is turned on and has completed its warm-up/ self-test cycle.
- Check the gas sample line for kinks, obstructions, etc.
- Ask the anesthesia provider if the ETT has moved or tilted.
- Check the circuit for disconnection or kinks.

Almost every gas analyzer problem I have been called about was remedied by a quick fix: changing the water trap and or changing the gas sample line. There is the rare occasion when the gas analyzer will be inadvertently cut off and then cut back on, which means it is cycling and we just have to wait.

Common CO2 Problems

- Elevated CO2 on the capnography.
- Replace the CO2 absorber.
- Examine inspiratory, and expiratory flow valves.
- Drain moisture from beneath the CO2 absorber

CAUSES OF ELEVATED $EtCO_2$	CAUSES OF DECREASED $EtCO_2$
METABOLISM Pain Hyperthermia Shivering	**METABOLISM** Hypothermia Metabolic acidosis
RESPIRATORY SYSTEM Respiratory insufficiency Respiratory depression COPD Analgesia/sedation	**RESPIRATORY SYSTEM** Alveolar hyperventilation Bronchospasm Mucus plugging
CIRCULATORY SYSTEM Increased cardiac output	**CIRCULATORY SYSTEM** Hypotension Sudden hypovolemia Cardiac arrest Pulmonary emboli
MEDICATIONS Bicarbonate administration	

Scavenging System

Overwhelmed scavenging system.

If there is a sound of escaping air into the room on expiration, do the following:

- Turn down the fresh gas flow.
- Check the vacuum control valve for proper adjustment.
- Check the gas disposal conduit.
- Check the disposal tubing for kinks.
- Always check the scavenger circuit for proper connection and for rips or holes.

Moisture in the anesthesia gas machine causes most of the malfunctions and errors and that's why I said at the beginning that proper and daily maintenance will greatly decrease errors.

Malignant Hyperthermia

Malignant Hyperthermia (MH) is a disease passed down through families that causes a fast rise in body temperature (fever) and severe muscle contractions when the affected person gets general anesthesia.

MH is a potentially fatal, inherited disorder usually associated with the administration of certain general anesthetics and or the drug succinylcholine. The disorder is due to an acceleration of metabolism in skeletal muscle.

SIGNS OF MH INCLUDE:

- Muscle rigidity
- Rapid heart rate
- High body temperature
- Muscle breakdown
- Increased acid content

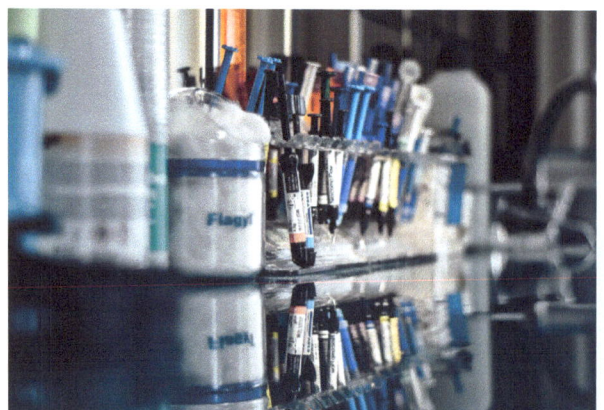

TREATMENT

Immediate treatment with the drug Dantrolene usually reverses the signs of MH. The underlying defect abnormally increases levels of cell calcium in the skeletal muscle.

There is mounting evidence that some patients will also develop MH with exercise and/or on exposure to hot environments. Without proper and prompt treatment with Dantrolene sodium, mortality is extremely high. The best way to protect yourself, your family, your patients, and the facility is to be prepared before it's too late. Make sure you are aware of your hospitals MH protocols.

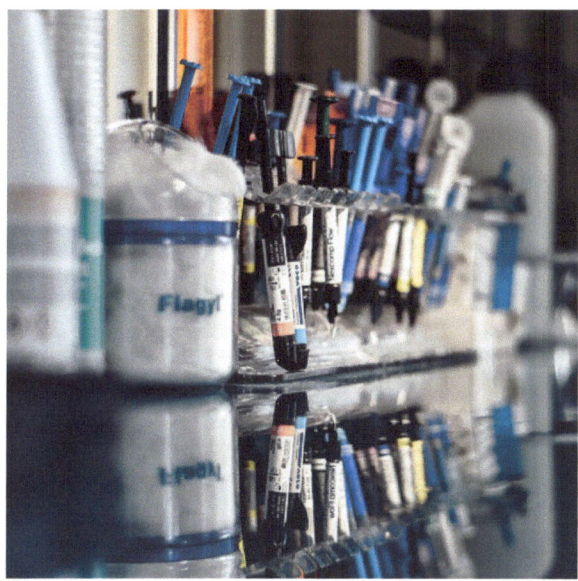

WHAT'S SHOULD BE IN EMERGENCY CART?

Medications

- Dantrolene – 36 vials
- Sterile preservative free water
- Sodium Bicarbonate 8.4% (50ml x 5)
- Furosemide (40mg/amp x 4 amps)
- Dextrose 50% (50ml vials x 2)
- Calcium Chloride 10% (10ml vial x 2)
- Regular Insulin (100 units x 1 refrigerated)
- Lidocaine preloaded syringes (100mg) x 3 or Amiodorone

Supplies

- Anesthesia circuit and sodasorb
- Temperature probe
- 60 cc syringes
- Mini-spikes
- Fluid transfer tubing
- N/G tube & Toomey syringes for irrigation
- Foley
- Zip baggies for ice packs
- Large bore IV's
- ICE & 3 Ls of cold IV and bottles saline in refrigerator

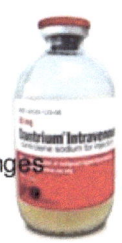

How to Prepare the Anesthesia Machine for MH Patients

Ensure that anesthetic vaporizers are disabled by removing or taping in the "OFF" position. **Most vaporizers have a significant reservoir of anesthetic that cannot be drained, thus draining is not an acceptable choice.**

Some Hotline consultants recommend changing CO_2 absorbent (soda lime or baralyme).

Flow 10 L/min O_2 through circuit via the ventilator for at least 20 minutes (refer to the consensus statement on page 36).

During this time, a disposable, unused breathing bag should be attached to the Y-piece of the circulation system and the ventilator set to inflate the bag periodically.

Use a new or disposable breathing circuit. Use the expired gas analyzer to conform the absence of volatile gasses, as some newer machines are not so easily cleaned of volatile agents.

Changing the CO_2 absorbent (soda lime or baralyme) is not recommended if these procedures are followed. Newer anesthesia "workstations" may require up to 104 minutes or more for purging residual gases; consult the

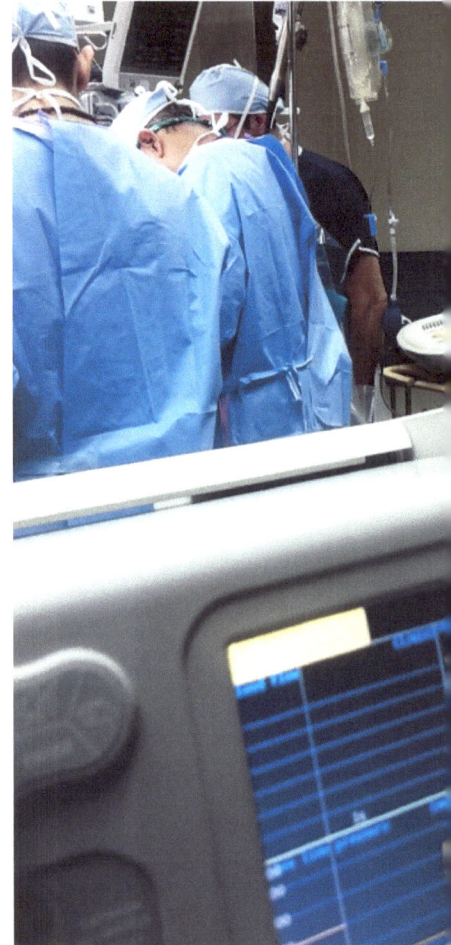

Adding commercially available charcoal filters to the circuit will remove anesthetic gases and therefore obviate the need for thorough purging the system as described. However, the anesthesia machine will still need to be flushed with high fresh gas flows for 90 seconds prior to placing the activated charcoal filters on the inspiratory and expiratory ports. These filters, when used in combination with a fresh gas flow of 10 lpm for the first 90 minutes with the option to reduce the flow rate to 3 lpm, may be effective for 12 hours.

ICU/Transport Bed Setup

A. Proper setup of a bed for transporting patients to the ICU:

1. You will need the following:

a. Transport monitor with modules for ECG, pulse ox, and 3 invasive pressure transducers; and a bundle of cables for all modules

> NOTE: Make sure the monitor battery is at least 50% charged. If any items are missing, inform the anesthesiologist and arrange a suitable plan (i.e., use modules from the OR).

b. O2 tank with at least 1000 PSI. Test the O2 flow to make sure the main valve on the tank is open and that O2 will flow.

c. Ambu-bag.

d. For cardiac rooms, a defibrillator that has been tested for sufficient battery power and has been test-fired within the previous 24 hours. e. IV pole on the appropriate side.

f. Some ICU bed setups require a defibrillator (ask a physician if one is required if unsure). All defibrillators should be checked for QCs (located on EKG printout) and should have a bottle of redux crème (electrolyte crème) taped to the back of the defibrillator.

2. Set the bed up as follows:

a. Make sure the bed is completely flat and has been set to the proper height (height of the OR table). If there is soiled linen or no linen, call the front desk and report this.

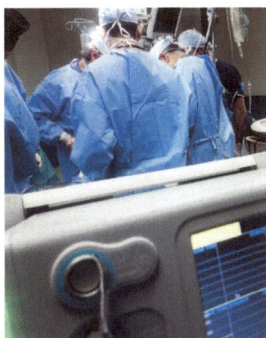

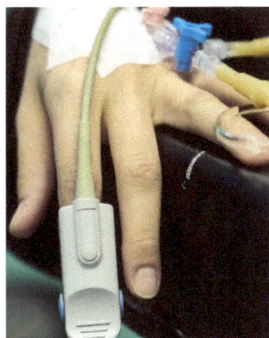

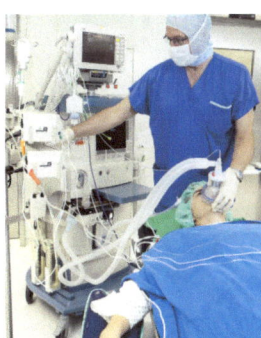

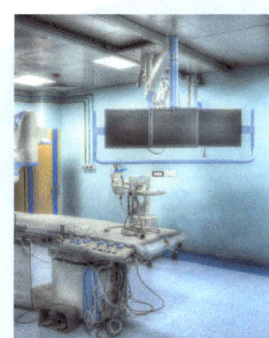

b. Position the O2 tank under the bed such that its regulator can be accessed when the bed has been taken into the room and pinned up against the OR bed in preparation for transferring the patient.

c. Place the monitor on the shelf at the foot of the bed. Strap it down, or tape it down if there is no strap present.

d. If the monitor is sitting for a while, disengage batteries from the monitor. Notify clinician to push batteries back in when ready to use the monitor.

e. Attach the cables to the monitor, and uncoil them, leaving them on the appropriate side of the bed (such that the patient will not be rolled over them when transferred).

f. Attach the ambu-bag's O2 line to the O2 tank regulator. Make sure the line is attached firmly. Save the mask that comes from the ambu-bag in a bag.

NOTE: If you are not certain that the ambu-bag will be used during the transport, do not remove it from the bag; just place it on the bed.

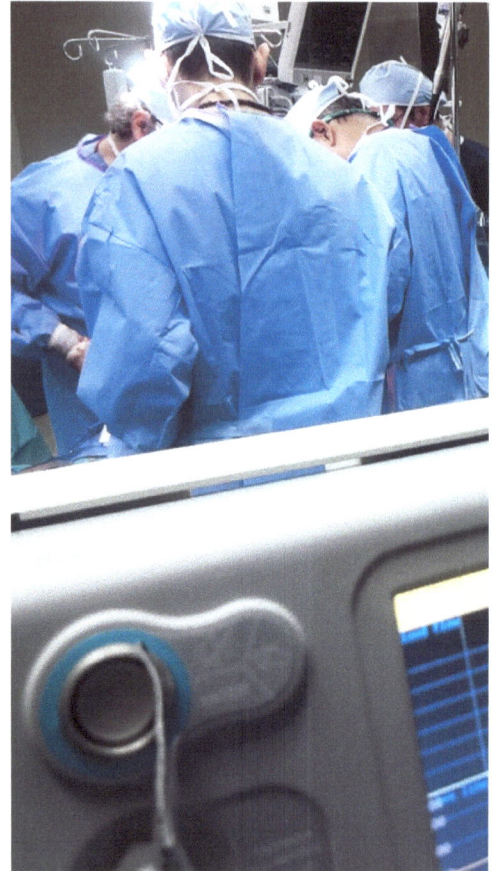

B. Notes:

- If the CLEANER's have not provided a proper bed promptly, it is some hospitals' protocol to leave the transport equipment on a cart outside the OR room, call the OR desk and request a bed, then return to set it up when it arrives.

-

- Some ICU beds do not have a shelf underneath for the O2 tank. In this case, you must provide a rack that clips to the head of the bed or nds some other means of properly restraining the tank.

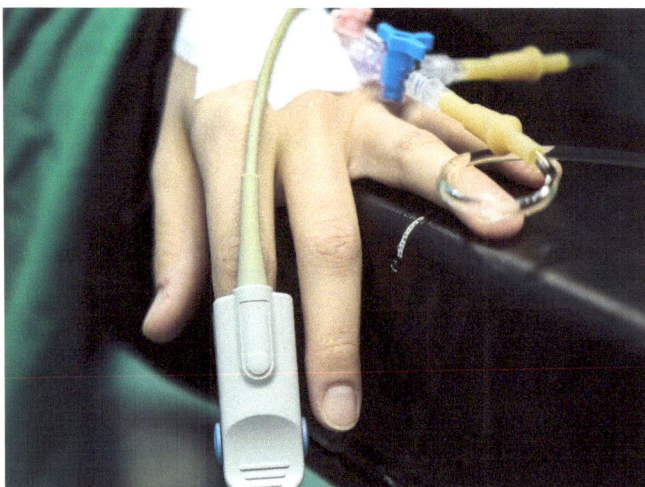

MRI Suite Precautions

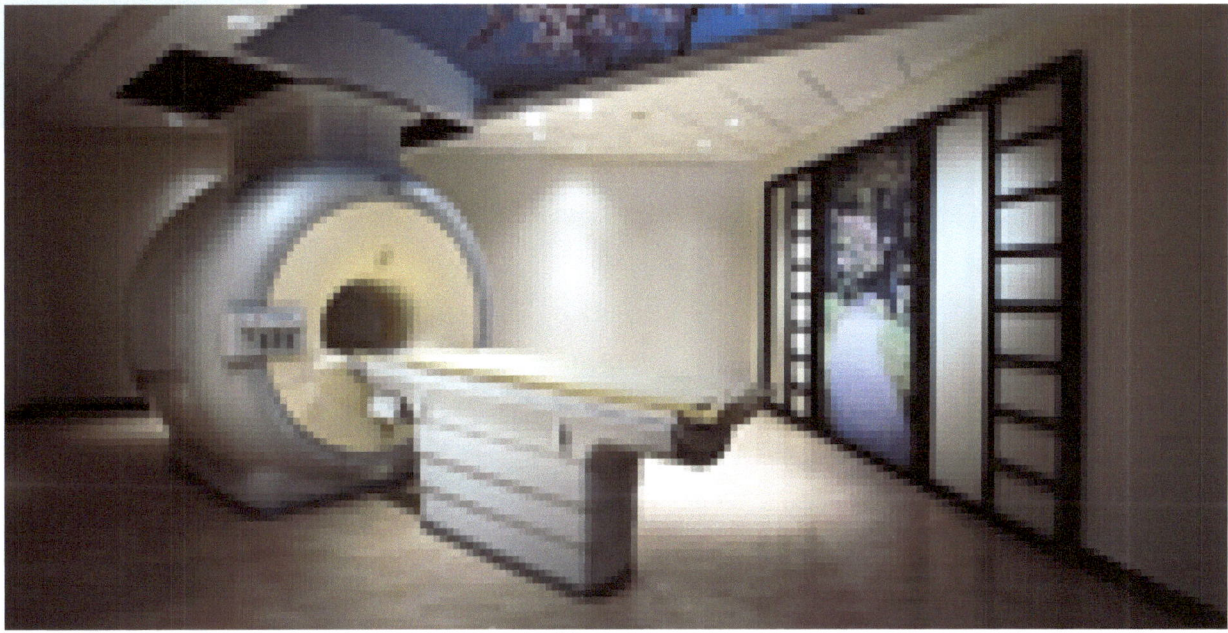

I. When dropping off the MRI supply cart:

- You MUST take the tank off the top of the cart and place it on an individual tank rack, or any place designated by MRI. This must be done in every circumstance, even if the MRI suites are closed and nobody is around, or even if the anesthesiologist and MRI employees are present.

- We must also remove the Baxter pump from the top of the MRI cart, making sure it stays outside of the suite.

When entering the MRI suites:

- If it is your first time entering the suites, you must find an MRI employee and respond to some important questions.
-
- If it is not your first time, you must alert the MRI techs that you are there and allow them to evaluate whether you have taken proper precautions for entering the suite.
-
- Remove all metal or magnetic objects you are carrying or wearing. This includes fanny packs, watches, IDs, etc.

INTERMEDIATE TRAINING

How to Build Invasive Pressure Transducers

Observe sterile techniques at all times.

Description:

To monitor real-time dynamic blood pressure and transfer it to signal processing systems for diagnosis, treatment and postoperative evaluation.
Compatible with all guardianship equipments.
Connectors available: Abbott,Utah,Edwards,BD,USB,B.Braun ISO&CE.

Pressure transducer kit includes:

— Transducer
— Infusion set
— Pressure monitoring line
— Stopcock
— Flushing Valve: 3ml/Adult, 30ml/Child
— Red,blue,yellow monitoring line is available

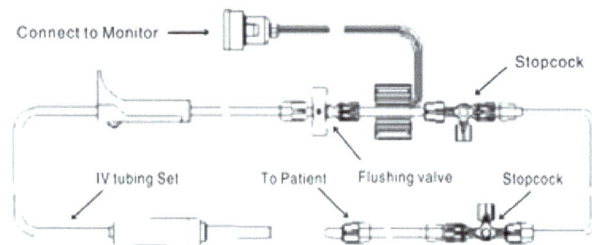

A. How to build and flush a transducer.

1. Find a transducer bracket and pole clamp set, and affix them to an IV pole.

2. Open your transducer set.

A) Briefly, unsnarl the tubing.
B) Place the transducer portion in its proper place on the bracket.
C) When making a triple transducer: Art-Line: Ensure to place the art-line transducer (color-coded red) in the leftmost bracket.
Put the CVP (central venous pressure) transducer (color coded blue) in the middle bracket. Put the PA (pulmonary artery) transducer (color coded yellow) in the rightmost bracket.
3. On all transducer lines, replace the distal female stopcock white cap (which has a hole in it) with a yellow or blue one (which is solid). Use sterile technique.

4. Tighten all connections.
5. Open a 500ml bag of. 9% NaCl and affix a label on it.
6. Fill in the date, time, and your initials.

7. Using sterile technique:

A) Invert the 500ml bag and spike it with the spike that is part of the transducer set.

B) With one hand, pull on the red pigtail of the transducer.

C) Using the other hand, gently squeeze the inverted 500 ml bag until all air is out of the bag and the drip chamber on the transducer's spike is filled with fluid.

8. Hang the bag on one of the loops of the IV pole.

9. With one hand, pull down on the transducer's pigtail allowing fluid from the bag to flush all portions of the tubing, including all stopcock ports. While inspecting the progress of the fluid through the tubing, making sure no air is left trapped. If any air is spotted, tap the tubing over it, keeping the pigtail open all the time, until it is dislodged and vented through the nearest port.

10. When you have finished flushing, close the distal stopcock to the transducer.

11. Place a 500ml pressure bag over the bag of NaCl and inflate to 300 PSI.

12. Close the stopcock on the pressure bag so that it maintains pressure

How to Install a Transducer

1. For each line on the transducer, take an invasive pressure module and cable.
2. In the OR, attach the transducer bracket to an IV pole.

NOTE:
Adjust the height of the transducer such that it will be the same height as the patient's heart when he/she is lying on the table during the surgery.

3. Place the modules in the module rack. Always place the module for the art-line in first, and position it the furthest left in the rack. The CVP should go in second, next to the art-line, and the PA last.

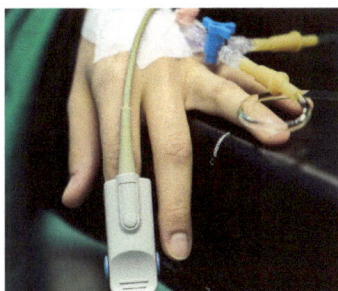

NOTE:
When setting up a double transducer set, the yellow line will be used for the arterial line and the blue for CVP.

4. Connect the art-line transducer to a cable, and plug the cable into the appropriate module. Do the same for any other transducers.

5. On the stopcock directly above the transducer portion, close the lever to the patient such that, if you were to flush the transducer, all the fluid would exit through the white cap on the stopcock.

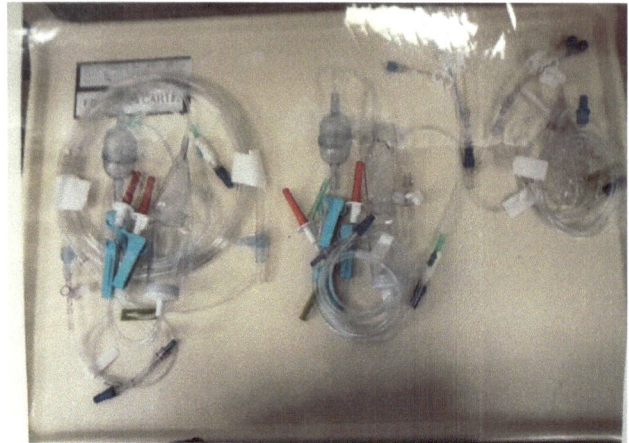

6. Press and hold the "zero" button on the pressure module until you hear a beep, or until you see, on the patient monitor, the message "art-line zero in the process."

7. Release the button on the module and wait until the monitor shows zero as the pressure reading for your transducer.

NOTE:
NOTE: Make sure you get the number "0" and that the number stays at 0 for a few seconds. If this does not occur, your zeroing process was not accepted or you have an equipment malfunction.

8. Re-open the line to the patient by turning the lever on the stopcock directly above the transducer to its original position. Ensure the monitor shows that pressure in the line goes up to approximately 300 psi.

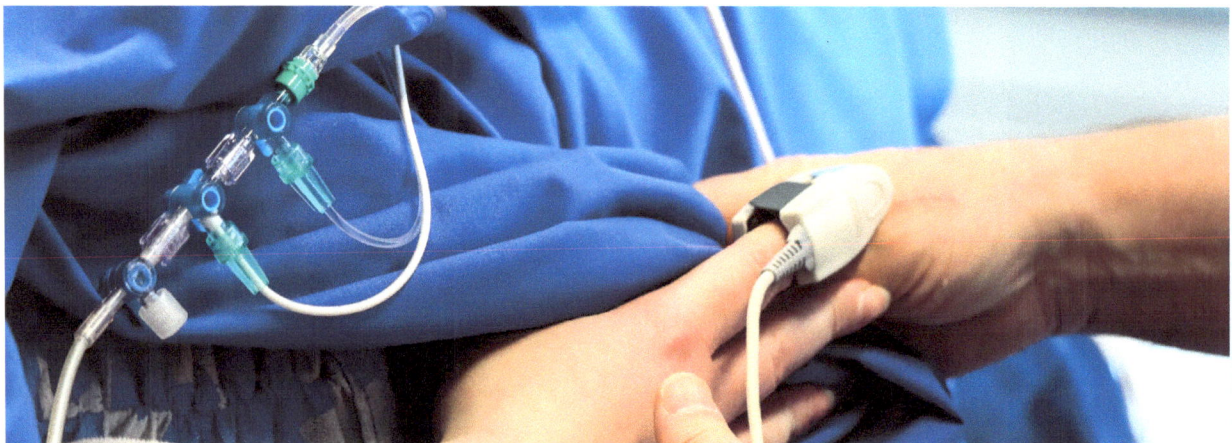

Setting Up the Level One

1. Tighten all connections on the Level One disposable warming set.

2. Insert the Level One disposable into the Level One. Make sure the air trap and water chamber are both pushed completely in.

3. Attach a wide bore (high-flow) stopcock to the end of the disposable tubing.

4. Attach a Level One extension set to the stopcock.

5. Hang all tubing, so it will not fall on the floor and is easily accessible.

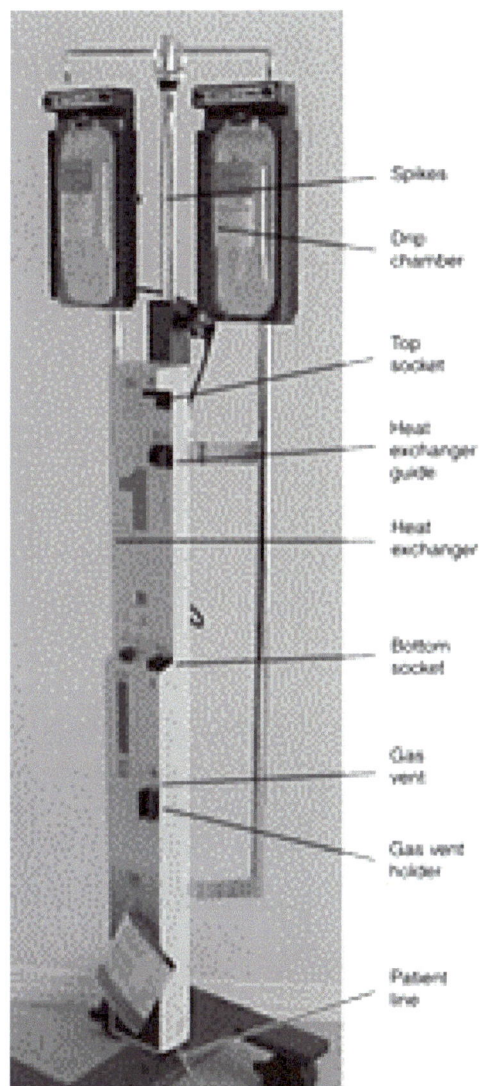

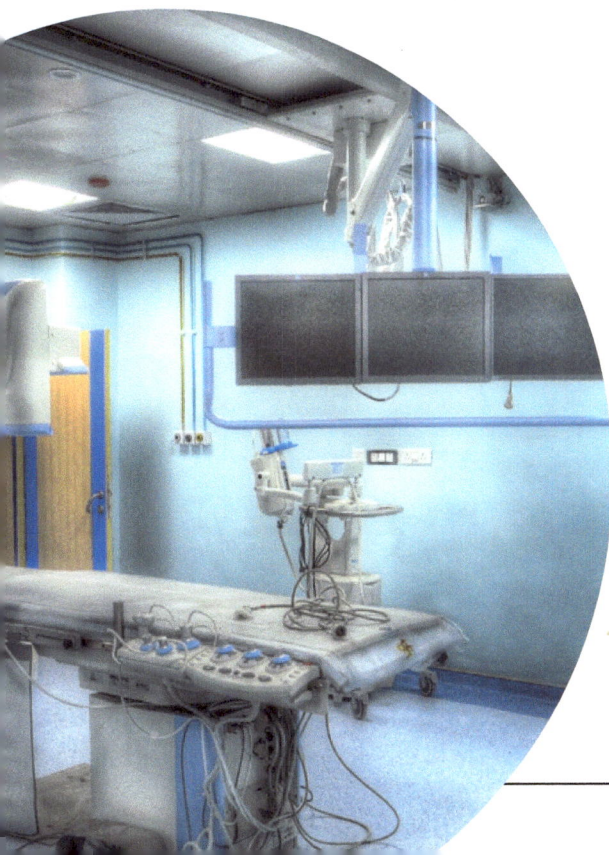

Spikes

Drip chamber

Top socket

Heat exchanger guide

Heat exchanger

Bottom socket

Gas vent

Gas vent holder

Patient line

Priming the Level One

1. Burp a 1-liter bag of normal saline (sodium chloride). **ALL FLUID MUST BE BURPED BEFORE ATTACHING TO THE LEVEL ONE. OTHERWISE, IT WILL PUSH THE AIR INTO THE PATIENT'S IV.**

2. Spike the normal saline (sodium chloride) bag and fill the drip chamber about halfway so that it is high enough to prevent air from getting in the tubing but low enough to easily see the drip rate.

3. Let line flush through, making sure all air bubbles have left the line.

4. Clamp IV using the main rolling clamp on the Level One disposable set.

5. Hang all tubing, so it will not fall on the floor and is easily accessible

Belmont Rapid Infuser Step-by-Step

The following is a step-by-step summary of the major steps; the remainder of the chapter explains each step in detail.

SETUP	
INSPECT THE SYSTEM • Power cord • Reservoir support • Disposable set • Large reservoir and holder, if needed	Inspect the system to ensure that you have all necessary components. Use only supplied power cord.

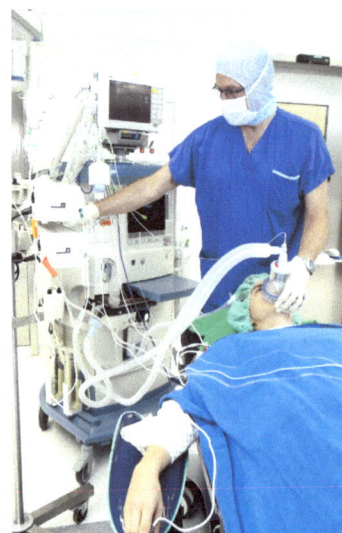

SETUP	

IV POLE MOUNTING

- IV pole: 5 wheel, maximum diameter 1 1/4"

- Install the support assembly 30" above the IV pole base Mount the F MS 2000 on the IV pole above the support assembly

- Install the reservoir support app. 9" above the top of the system

CAUTION: Check that the system is securely clamped to an IV pole and will not tip over

1. Install the support assembly (support clamp and washer) approximately 30" from IV pole base.

While holding clamp closed, loosen the screw to open up the clamp. Install clamp on the IV pole, holding clamp close and tighten screw using supplied 3/16 Allen wrench. Snap the plastic washer onto the IV pole above the support clamp.

2. Lift up on the "Pole Clamp Release Handle" to open mount the system on the IV pole above the support system by pushing down on the pole clamp release handle. Check that the system is locked in place before proceeding.

3. Clamp the reservoir support onto the IV pole approximately 9" above the F MS 2000. •

- Make certain that there is nothing obstructing the air vents at the bottom of the system.

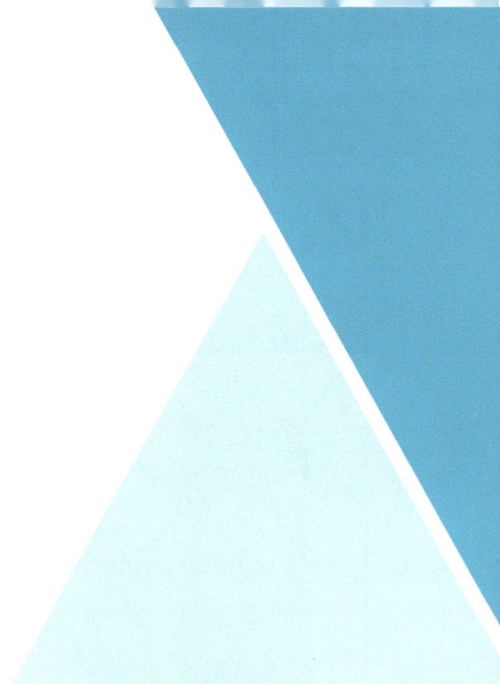

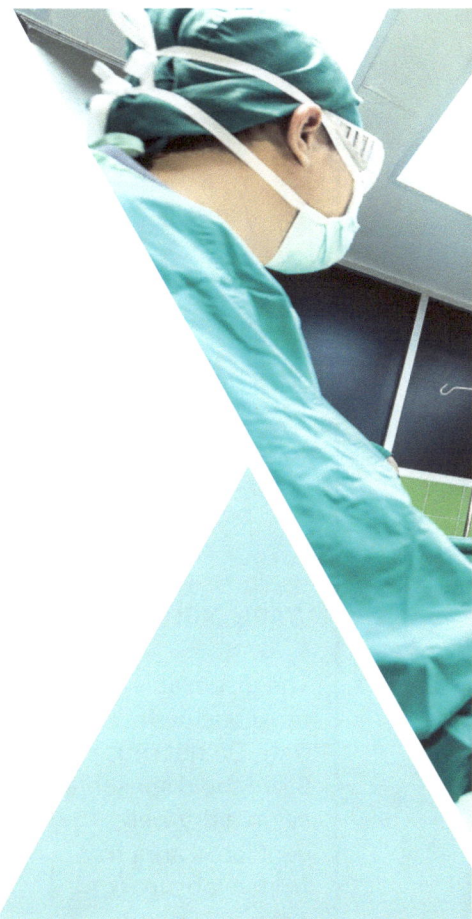

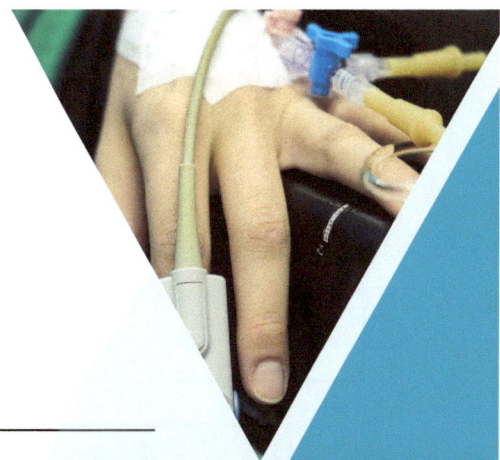

SETUP	

INSTALLING DISPOSABLE SET 3- Spike Disposable set with key components
 	
 WARNING:
 	
 The disposable set is for single patient use only. Do not reuse. Store the disposable set in a dry well ventilated area free from exposure to chemical vapors. Always apply first-in, first-out technique to minimize the length of storage for any unit.
	1. Snap reservoir chamber into the reservoir support clamp.
	
	  2. Open the door. Insert heat exchanger with red arrow pointing up (Red tinted tubing to red stripe on unit)
	
	  3. Firmly position the interlock into the fluid out detector.
	
	 4. Guide the curved piece of pump tubing (Blue tinted tubing) over the pump head. Check that the thinner recirculate line is in the grove to the right.
	
	 Do not kink or twist the tubing.
	
	  5. Place the pressure chamber into the pressure chamber well. Firmly insert the wider infuse line into the air detector and to the left of valve wand.
	
	 Do not apply excessive pressure to the pressure transducer. The pressure transducer can be damaged with excessive force. Do not use the system if the pressure transducer is damaged.
	
	 6. Place the thinner recirculate line to the right of the air detector, and to the right of the valve wand.
	
	 7. Close and latch the door. Make certain the pump tubing is not caught. Connect the patient line.

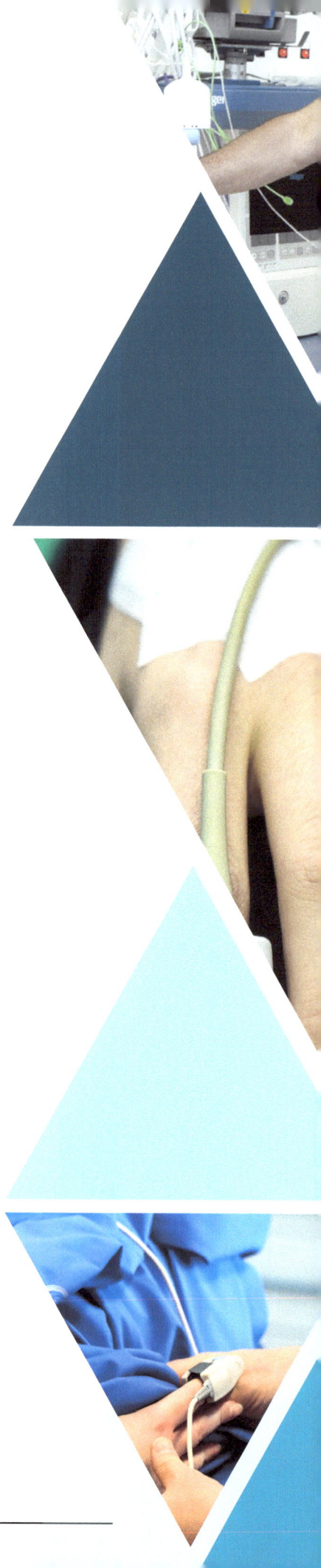

SETUP

INSTALL LARGE RESERVOIR, IF NEEDED

- Install the large reservoir holder

- Install large reservoir

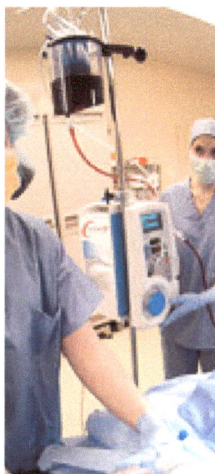

CAUTION:

Do not pressurize or apply a vacuum to the reservoir

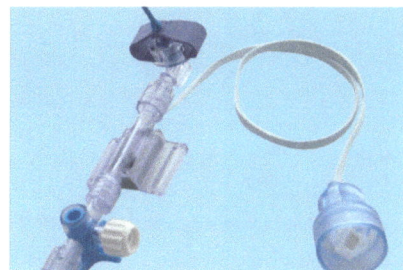

1. Using aseptic techniques, remove the reservoir chamber from the 3-spike disposable set by disconnecting the Luer connectors. • Disconnect the larger pump tubing by pressing in the Luer lock tab and pulling out the connector.
• Disconnect the thinner recirculate line by unscrewing the connector.

2. Attach the reservoir holder onto the IV pole and place the reservoir into the holder.

3. Assemble the large reservoir using aseptic techniques by attaching the three fluid supply tails onto the top of the reservoir.

4. Connect the large reservoir to the Luer of the 3-spike disposable set.

5. Adjust the reservoir holder to make sure that the two connection leads underneath the reservoir are not stretched or kinked.

6. Stretched or kinked connection leads can cause flow restrictions and frequent fluid-out alarms.

Install the 3-spike disposable set into the F MS 2000, as previously shown.

SETUP	
POWER ON Check that the detachable power cable is securely seated in the main power receptacle. Plug the system power cord into a grounded, 3-prong, 20 amps, AC receptacle. Do not use an adaptor for ungrounded outlets.	Turn power on by firmly pressing the circuit breaker to the ON position. The system will perform a self-check to check the integrity of system parameters. AC POWER PRESENT appears at the logo screen when the system first powers up. Check the power cord and AC receptacle connections if the statement does not appear. PRIME screen will appear. If you turn power ON without the disposable set, MISSING DISPOSABLE message and alarm will appear. Open the door or press MUTE to silence the alarm then install the disposable set as described earlier. Press NEXT to go to the PRIME screen.

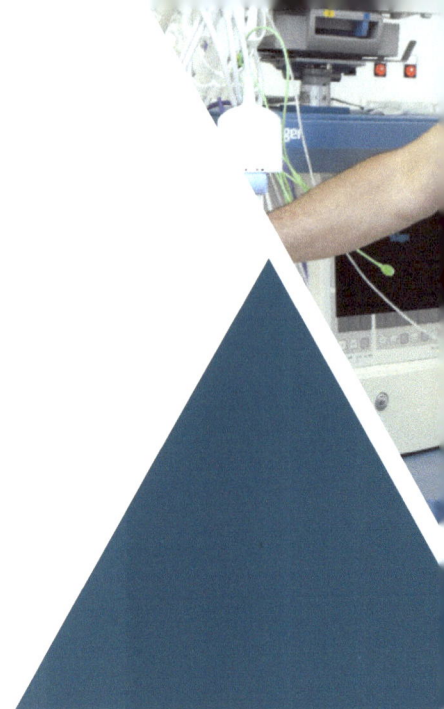

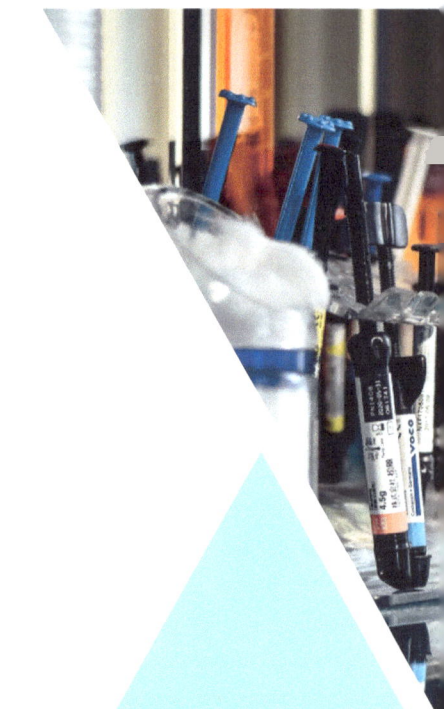

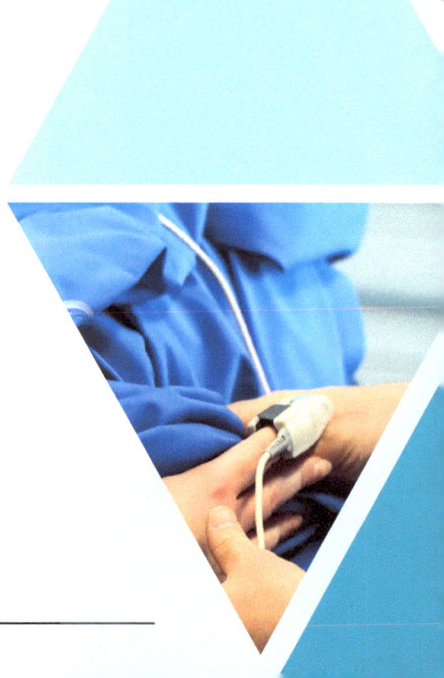

SETUP	
INSTALLING FLUID BAG Install solution compatible with blood for the main system prime.	Hang fluid bag on the IV pole. Close bag clamps, remove the bag spike cap(s). Spike fluid bag(s), pierce it fully to ensure that fluids flow freely. Open bag clamps. When hanging the fluid bag above the machine, the pump tubing that is seated in the fluid out detector should not be stretched. Stretching the pump tubing may cause false fluid-out alarms. The recirculate line must not be kinked or restricted.

SETUP	
PRIME THE MAIN SYSTEM Prime the main system with solution compatible with blood. Do not prime with blood.	1. Press PRIME to recirculate 100 ml of fluid at 500 ml/min to remove air and replace the main system with fluid. 2. The prime volume, 100 ml, countdown is displayed on the screen. Stop automatically when countdown reaches 0 ml. 3. If after 30 seconds the prime volume remains at 100 ml, the system will stop, alarm and instruct the user to unclamp the lines and resume prime. 4. If prime has to be stopped, press STOP. The prime volume countdown will remain on the screen. Press RESUME PRIME to continue prime.

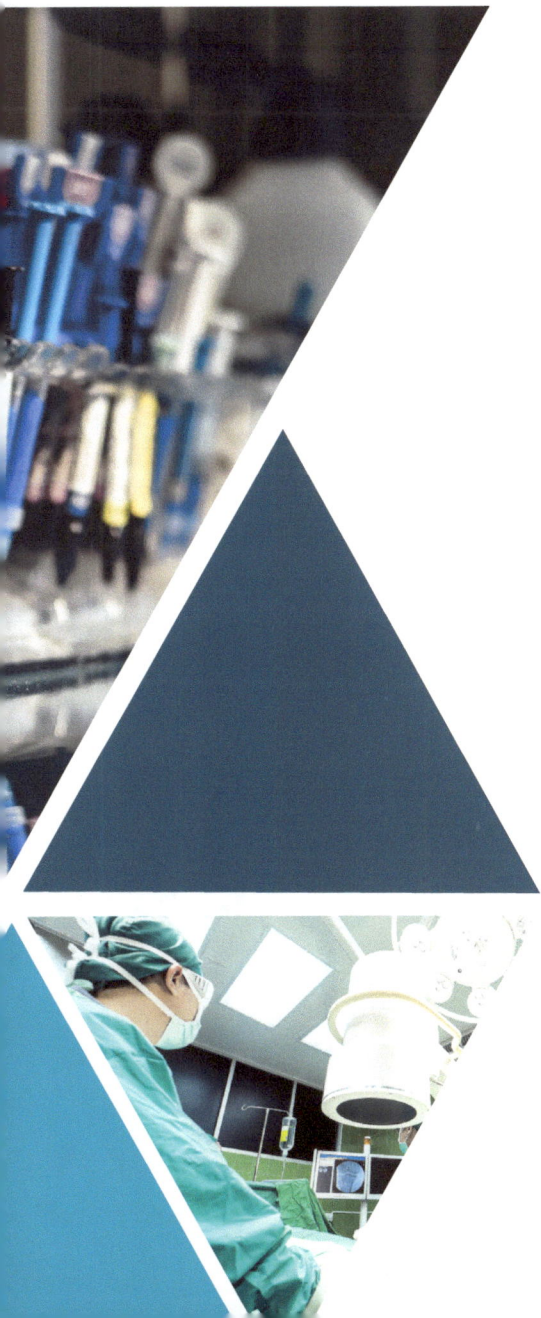

SETUP

PRIME THE PATIENT LINE

To remove air from the patient line.

WARNING!

Before continuing, you must inspect and make certain that the patient line is completely primed and free of air. Any air bubbles after the diversion valve in the patient line must be removed before the procedure can safely continue.

1. Open the roller clamp and remove the Luer cap.

2. Press PT. LINE PRIME Press once, prime at 50 ml/min. Press and hold, prime at 200 ml/min.

3. Press STOP after no air in patient line. Inspect to make sure that no air in the patient line. If there are air bubbles after the diversion valve, press PT. LINE PRIME to remove air.

SETUP

CONNECT TO THE PATIENT

Match infusion set to flow rate and fluid type, see chart.

1. Select an appropriate cannula size for decided flow rate.

2. Using aseptic technique, make patient connections without entrapping air

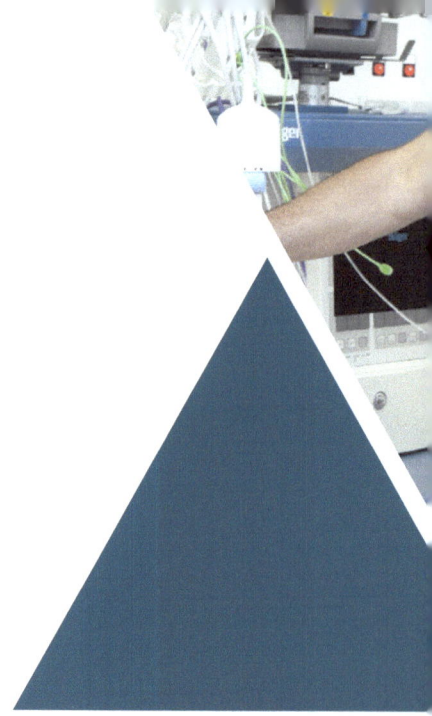

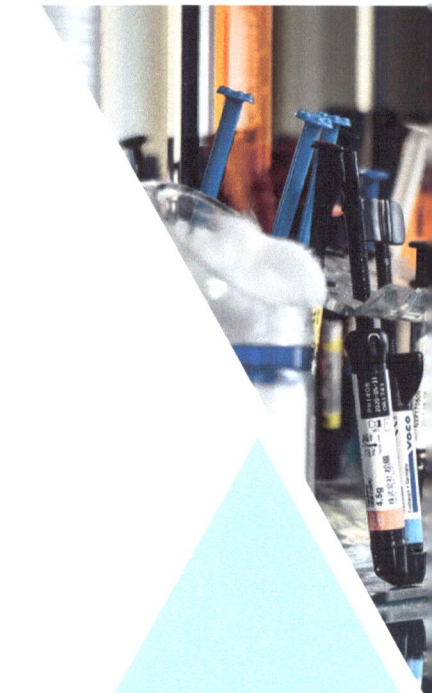

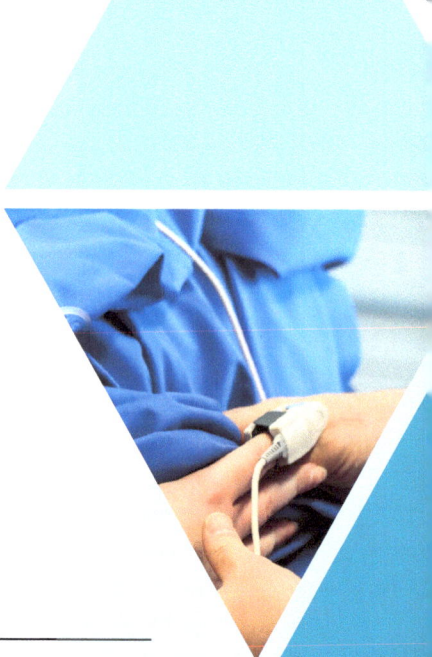

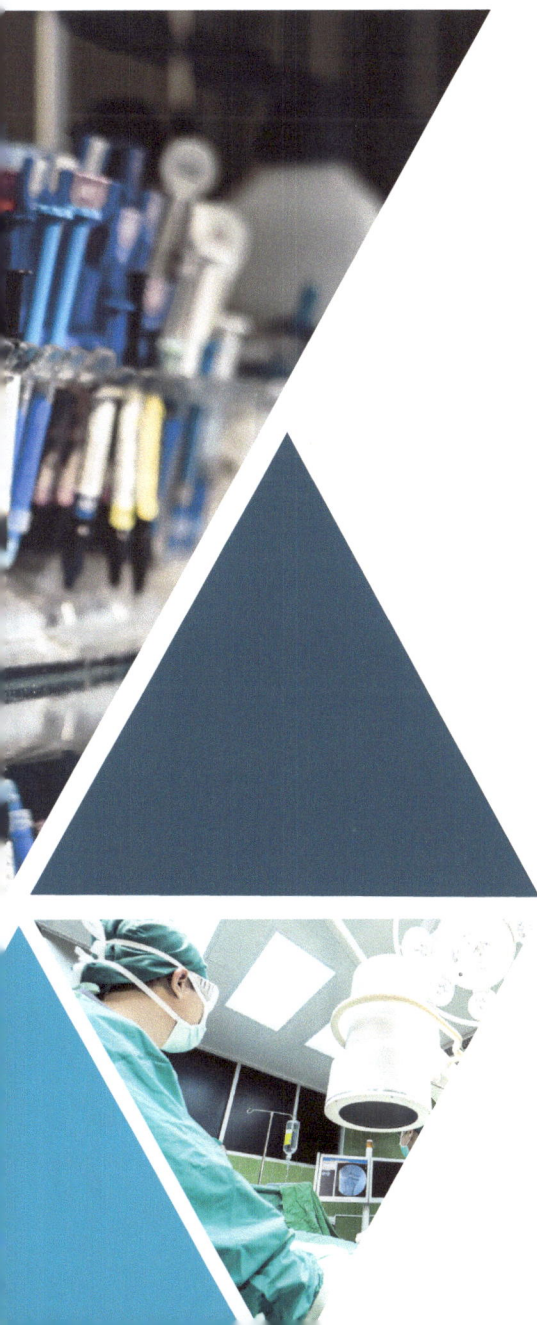

SETUP

INITIATING INFUSION

WARNING:

Do not mix lactated Ringer's or other solution containing calcium with citrated blood products Use only anticoagulated blood products

1. Press INFUSE to start infusing at 10 ml/min.

2. Press, 500 ML/MIN key to infuse at 500 ml/min or adjust flow rate, as needed, by pressing INFUSE RATE /INFUSE RATE key.

There is no heat at 2.5 and 5.0 ml/min settings. The message "LOW FLOW, NO HEAT" flashing on the screen indicates that the system is not heating at low flow rates.

SETUP

MAINTAIN INFUSION

CAUTION:

Replace reservoir chamber or disposable set every 4 hours or less when blood products are used to limit bacterial growth and maintain proper flow.

< Pressure Control

Regulate the pump speed to keep line pressure under the user-set pressure limit.

Routinely check patient and system parameters, on screen. Respond to and correct system alarms.

"The filter traps cells, cellular debris, and coagulated protein, resulting in a high protein concentration at the filter surface" (AABB 13th Edition)*. * American Association of Blood Banks, Technical Manual 13th Edition

The pressure status line flashes and a periodic beep sounds while the system is under pressure control. Line pressure is mainly due to the small orifice of the infusion set or any occlusions in the line.

The pressure limit is set at the factory to the maximum limit of 300 mmHg. To reduce the limit, Parameters Set-Up.P

SETUP	
< Automatic Air Purging **Remove air from the main system.**	After every 500 ml of fluid infused, the system automatically purges air from the system. The RATE status line displays REMOVING AIR during this process. The volume readout (VOL) remains unchanged during automatic air purging and resumes counting when the infusion resumes. The recirculate rate is temporarily set to 500 ml/min during automatic air purging, if the flow rate is at or below 500 ml/min. The recirculate rate is at the actual flow rate, if the flow rate is above 500 ml/min. When infusion resumes, the system returns to the previously set rate.
< Bolus **Deliver fixed volume at a rate of 200 ml/min.**	The bolus volume is set at the factory to 200 ml. This can be changed in the Parameters Set-Up screen or by pressing and holding the BOLUS key in the Infuse screen. The new bolus volume will appear in the VOL (volume) status line with the prefix of BOL (bolus). Releasing the Bolus key will start the infusion. To change the flow rate during the bolus infusion, press the INFUSE RATE or INFUSE RATE or 500 ml/min RATE key. Two sets of numbers are displayed within the BOLUS key space. The top number is the bolus value set and the bottom number is the volume pumped and is counting up from 0 to the volume set on the key. At the end of the bolus volume, the system beeps and returns to the previously selected flow rate if the previous rate was 50 ml/min or lower. If the previous rate was higher than 50 ml/min, the flow rate will be set to 50 ml/min.

SETUP	
BATTERY OPERATION **(NO HEAT)**	1. Press RECIRC key to preheat fluid in the reservoir chamber. 2. Unplug the system from the wall outlet. The status line that displays temperature will be flashing BATTERY NO HEATING to indicate the system is now in battery mode, the maximum flow rate is 50 ml/min, and heating is suspended. 3. Adjust the flow rate by pressing INFUSE RATE or INFUSE RATE or press 50 ML/MIN to immediately set the infuse rate to the maximum rate of 50 ml/min. 4. When the system is plugged back to the AC outlet, the flow rate stays at 50 ml/min if the previous flow rate was greater than 50 ml/min. The system will return to the previous flow rate if the previous rate was 50 ml/min or lower. 5. The normal running time in battery is at least 30 minutes.

SETUP	
END OF PROCEDURE Before opening the door, clamp the patient line closed.	1. Clamp off patient line and bag spikes. 2. Turn circuit breaker to STANDBY. 3. Remove disposable set and dispose in according to the hospital policy. 4. Clean and disinfect the system.

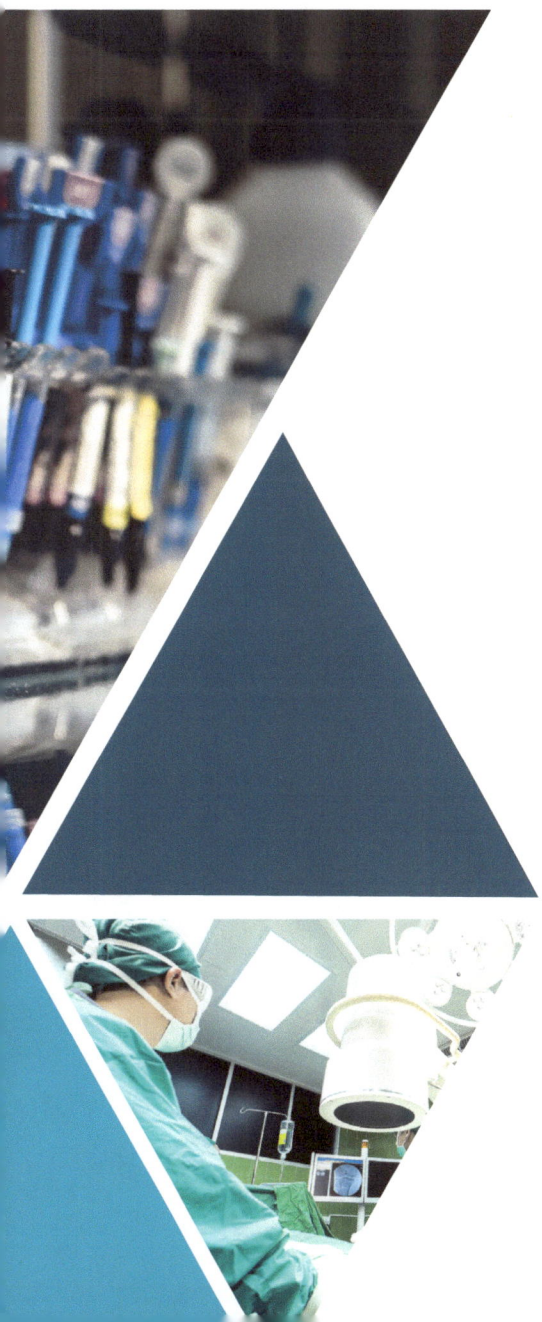

Thermacor 1200 Assembly

1. Load the disposable cassette.

2. Put the large fluid volume reservoir inside of its ring holder.

3. Connect the larger fluid volume reservoir with the disposable cassette via the bundled tubing to the blue covered connector on the disposable cassette.

4. Connect the dual patient line to the red-covered connector on the disposable cassette.

5. Attach two high-flow stopcocks to the ends of the dual patient line.

6. Attach two level-one extensions to the high-flow stopcocks.

7. Connect the ends of the level-one extensions to the Luer-lock openings of the large fluid volume reservoir.

8. Connect the return line to the yellow connector (air vent line).

9. Prime the reservoir with 1L of Normal Saline. See Attached Quick Reference Guide for instructions on how to operate the Thermacor.

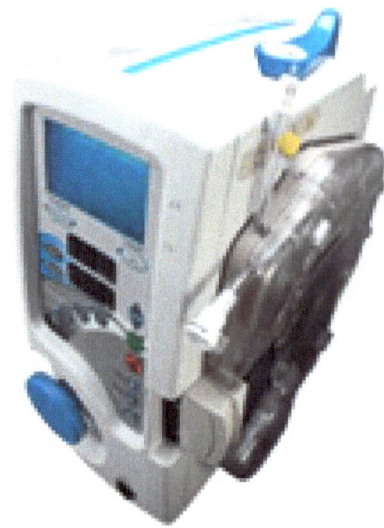

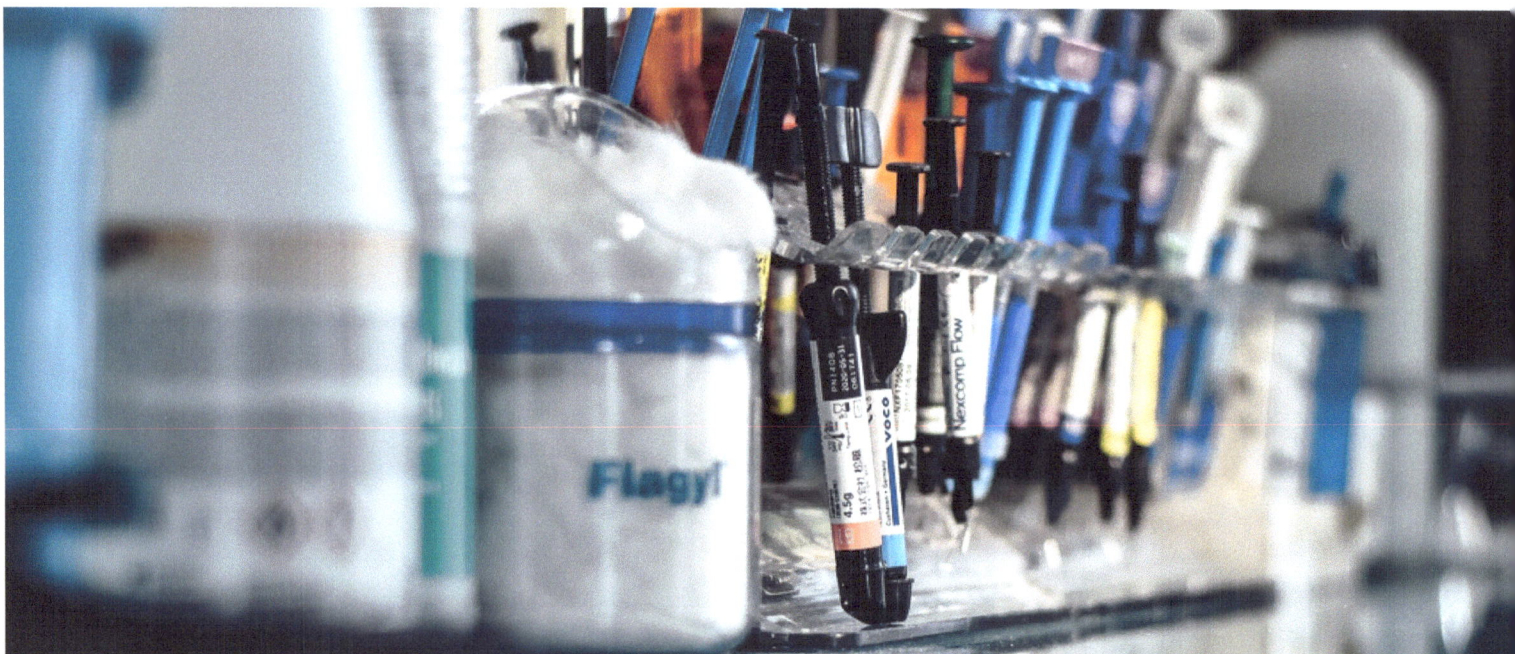

Building and Flushing a Standard IV Line

Observe sterile techniques at all times.

1. Attach a stopcock with extension set (walrus tubing) to a macro drip primary IV set.

2. Hang a 1-liter bag of LR (or normal saline/sodium chloride) and spike with the primary IV set.

3. Squeeze the drip chamber and allow it to fill roughly halfway, which is high enough to prevent air from starting in the tubing but low enough to easily watch the trickle rate.

4. Let the line flush through, making sure all air bubbles have escaped the line.

5. Clamp IV using the rolling clamp on the primary IV set.

Standard IV Line While Using a Blood Warmer

Observe sterile technique at all times. 1. Insert Ranger fluid warmer disposable in Ranger fluid warmer.

2. Attach the Y-type blood set to the inside of the Ranger disposable.

3. Attach a stopcock with extension set (walrus tubing) to the outside of the Ranger disposable.

4. Hang a 1-liter bag of normal saline (sodium chloride) and spike with one side of the Y-type blood set (be sure the other spike is clamped off before spiking normal saline/sodium chloride).

5. Squeeze the drip chamber and allow it to fill about halfway, which is high enough to prevent air from getting in the tubing but low enough to easily see the drip rate.

6. Let the line flush through the Ranger disposable.

7. Inver the air trap on the outside of the Ranger disposable and allow it to fill completely with normal saline (sodium chloride).

8. Turn the air trap right side up and place in its holder.

9. Let the line flush through the rest of the tubing, making sure all air bubbles have left the line.

10. Clamp IV using the main rolling clamp on the Y-type blood set.

_____

ADVANCE TRAINING

Blood Draws from Transducer

Arterial Line Transducer

1. Attach a 10-ml Luer-lock syringe to the access port on the transducer and turn the stopcock to connect the syringe to the patient line.

2. Draw 10ml worth of fluid into the syringe.

3. Turn the stopcock to a 45-degree angle and remove the syringe (save or discard, depending on preference).

4. Connect sample/blood gas syringe and draw the specified amount of blood. Now repeat step 3.

5. Turn the stopcock to allow access to the Pressure bag.

6. Flush transducer with a gauze pad covering the access port. (Pull the blue pigtail to flush.) Cap off access port.

7. Turn the stopcock to connect the patient line with pressure bag.

8. Flush patient line until blood is no longer visible.

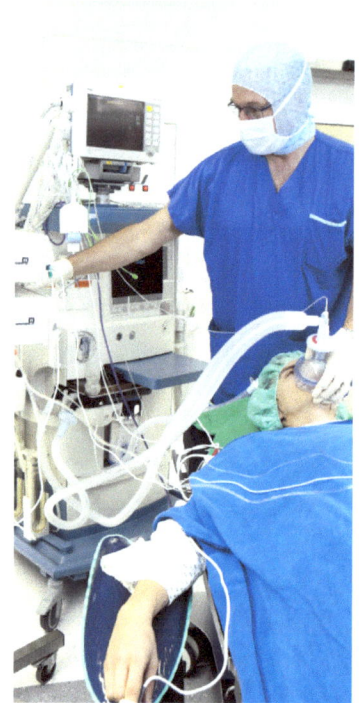

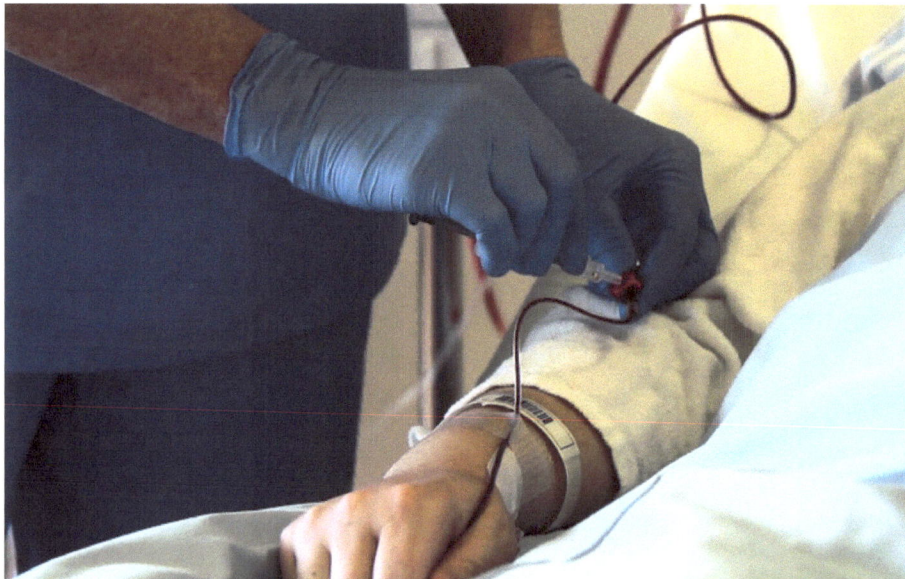

_____

Regional Anesthesia

Regional anesthesia is the technique of rendering a portion of a patient's body insensate to surgical stimuli. A patient may be having surgery on a part of the body, such as the hand, foot or shoulder, and not even realize that the operation is occurring! This is accomplished by placing a local anesthetic medication (the "-caine" drugs) near the nerves that go to that portion of the body. Examples of regional blocks include spinal, epidurals or peripheral nerve blocks.

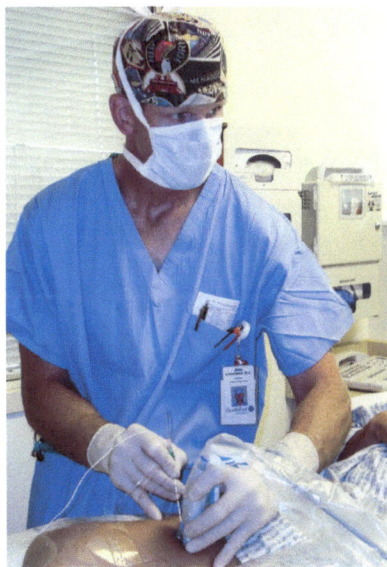

Equipment

Equipment needed includes the following: ANESTHESIA TECHNICIAN SURVIVAL GUIDE TPANG

- Ultrasound machine with linear transducer (8-14 MHz)
- Sterile sleeve
- Gel (or another coupling medium; e.g., normal saline/sodium chloride)
- Standard nerve block tray
- 20 to 25 ml local anesthetic
- 5-cm, 22-gauge short-bevel insulated stimulating needle
- Peripheral nerve stimulator - Sterile gloves

Setting Up the Cell-Saver

Observe sterile technique at all times.

1. Get a cell-saver bowl set and write down the information required on the cell-saver sheet. Hang a clipboard with the cell-saver sheet on the top hook of the cell-saver pole.

2. Insert the cell-saver bowl set into the cell-saver. Make sure the bowl is seated completely and tubing is placed properly in pump and valve.

3. Attach the waste bag to the cell-saver and connect it to the bowl set.

4. Hang collection bag on the top hook of the cell-saver pole.

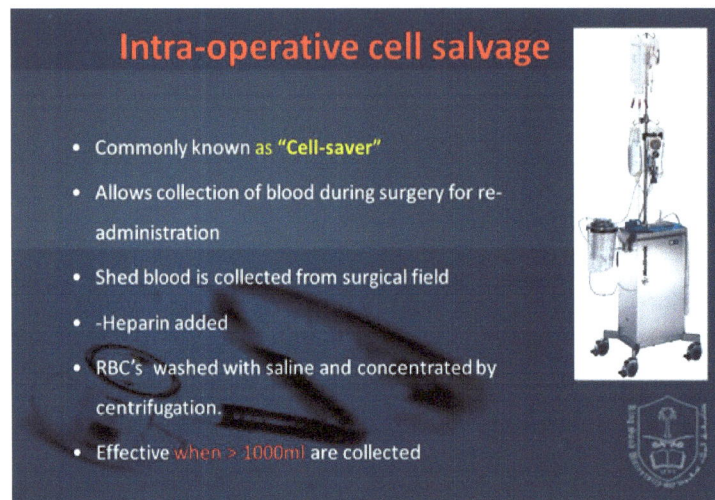

5. Hang two 1-liter normal saline (sodium chloride) bags on the lower hook of the cell-saver pole. Do not spike the normal saline (sodium chloride) bags.

6. Place reservoir in the holder. The bowl set should not be hooked up to the tubing from the reservoir until it is reasonably certain there is or will be enough blood to make a full bowl.

7. Clamp tubing on the bottom of the reservoir. Make sure it is completely clamped.

8. Make sure the cell-saver has the following with it:

   A. A properly set up bowl kit and reservoir.

   B. Unopened suction tubing.

   C. Two bags of normal saline (un-spiked) hanging on a lower hook of the IV pole.

   D. A clipboard holding paperwork with disposable kit information filled out.

   E. A bucket containing four 300 ml blood collection bags, two 600 ml collection bags, Pall filter, clips, scissors, and a clamp.

9. As a time saver, in an emergency, bring into the room and hook up the reservoir and suction setup to the heparinized saline. The rest of the cell-saver can be set up after the suction tubing has been attached.

How to Deliver the Cell-saver into the Operating Room

Observe sterile technique at all times.

1. 1-liter bag of heparinized normal saline. Be sure the cell-saver has the following with it BEFORE you bring it to a room:

2. A properly set up bowl kit and reservoir.

    a. Unopened suction tubing.

    b. Heparinized bag of saline hanging on an upper hook of the IV pole.

    c. Two un-spiked bags of normal saline (sodium chloride) hanging on a lower hook of the IV pole.

    d. A clipboard holding paperwork with disposable kit information filled out.

    e. A bucket containing four 300 ml blood collection bags, two 600 ml collection bags, Pall filter, clips, scissors, and a clamp. Bring cell-saver into the room.

3. Give circulation nurse unopened suction tubing. 4. Place cell-saver on the side of the room it will be set up on.

Establishing the Suction

(YOU NEED A REGULATOR)

Observe sterile technique at all times.

1. The vacuum level should be set to 150 mm Hg by doing the following:

a. Turn suction on.

b. Put a thumb over the metal port on the suction trap, or pinch off tubing leading from the metal port on the suction trap.

c. Increase or decrease adjustment knob as needed to set the dial to 150

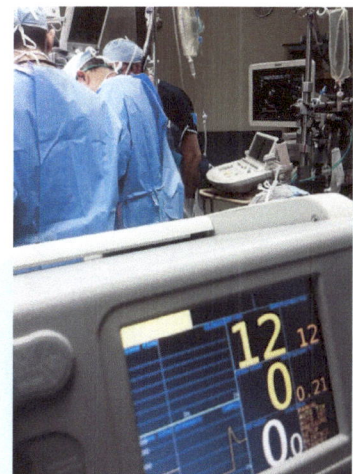

2. Hook the table-suction line to the blue port on the top of the reservoir first. The white port should be used as a backup.

3. Spike the heparinized saline bag with the spike on the suction tubing. Bring down 100 ML of anticoagulant to the reservoir at the beginning of the case when first hooking up the suction and also at any time you have emptied it.

4. The anticoagulant drip rate should be a minimum of 1 drop per second or greater depending on the quantity of blood being collected. Target ratio is approx. 100 ml of heparinized saline for every 700-ml of whole blood. In cases of very heavy blood loss, the drip rate should be set at whatever it takes to keep the blood from clotting off the bottom of the reservoir.

5. Fill out the paperwork. If you set up the suction in the case, you are responsible for filling out the heading on the paperwork (patient name, ID, surgeon, etc.).

Suction can be established from the wall suction or the internal vacuum of the cell-saver; however, it rst must pass through the regulator before reaching the reservoir.

Advanced Cell-Saver

Once you are comfortable with setting up and running the cell-saver, you might run into some uncomfortable situations. For example, the reservoir may overfill because the blood loss from the patient is too rapid. Also, you might be asked to wash blood cells that have been brought down from the blood bank.

In the former case, you might be inclined to bring a second (or third) cell-saver into the room. This will work but takes much more effort in managing. A good alternative is to have a second reservoir attached to the first reservoir, effectively doubling the amount of blood you can collect while the cell-saver is spinning blood.

For this you will need:

1. Second IV pole

2. Reservoir clamp holder

3. Second reservoir

4. Either a Y-type or single blood set

Attach the Luer-lock male end of the blood set to the vertical female end of the first cell-saver reservoir. Spike the tubing on the bottom of the second reservoir, which should be held in place in the clamp on the extra IV pole.

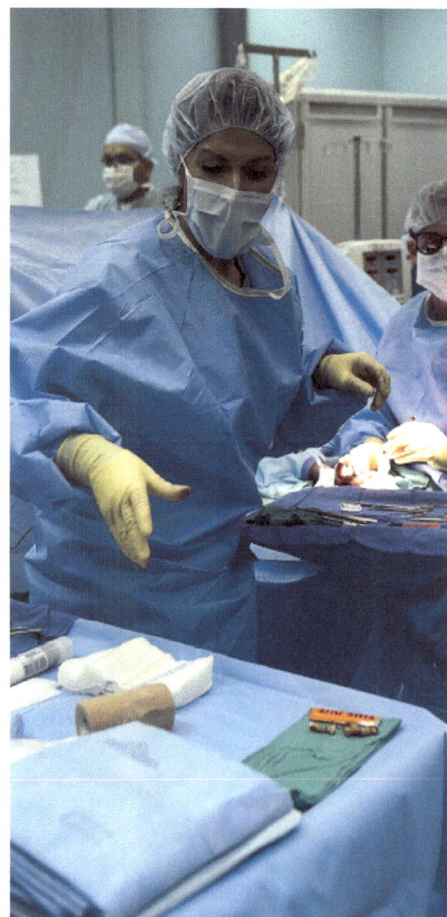

Washing Red Blood Cells

For this you will need:

1. Second cell-saver

Connect the blood set to the canister and spike the blood; wash as necessary. This removes excess electrolytes, such as potassium, from the blood product that the clinician does not want to introduce to the patient during transfusion

Waste Bag Full

If the waste bag fills up, the cell-saver will stop spinning. You should empty the waste bag at this point. To do this:

- Connect one end of the suction tubing to the exit port on the bottom of the waste bag.

- Ask the nurse in the room to connect the other end to the Neptune.

- Open the port and the waste will empty into the Neptune.

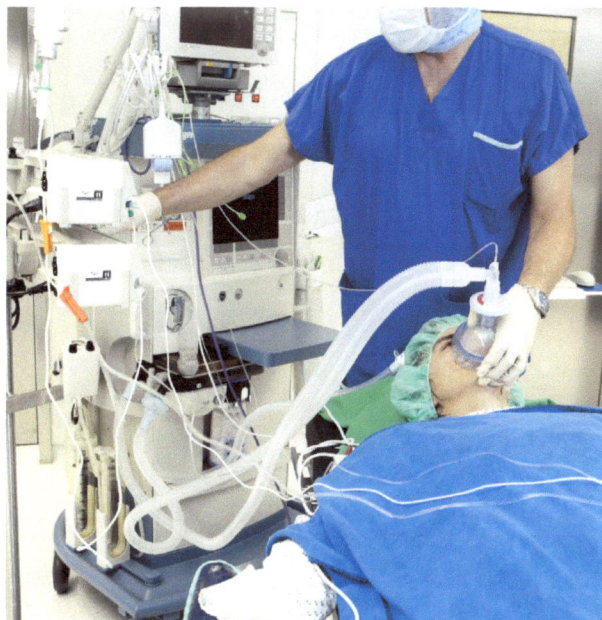

Cell-Saver Centrifuge Cleaning Mode

- Hold the green button when turning on the cell-saver to access this mode.

- Put a pink bucket under the cell-saver.

- Pour 70 isopropyl alcohol in the centrifuge. This will run through the inside of the machine and wash out any dried blood.

Using Wall Vacuum Suction

**Connect one end of the suction tubing to a white vacuum quickconnect and the other end to the regulator on the cell-saver. **

If you do this improperly, you can potentially suck blood into the wall vacuum system.

Trauma Room Setup

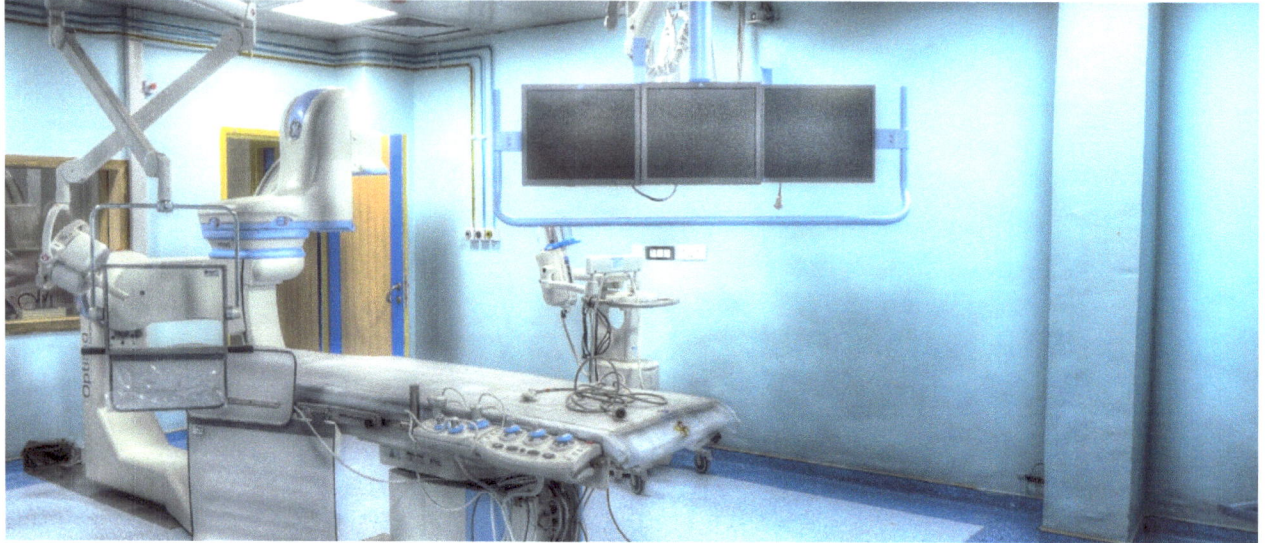

- Bair hugger
- Ranger fluid warmer
- Chair (one anesthesia chair per operating room)
- Isoflurane vaporizer

The following modules with cables:

  - EKG - Pulse ox

  - Noninvasive blood pressure

  - Temperature box

- Pressure lines: Double or triple transducer based on anesthesia provider/resident preference
- Tube tree
- BIS monitor
- Trauma carts – Baxter x 2
- Level one – dry setup

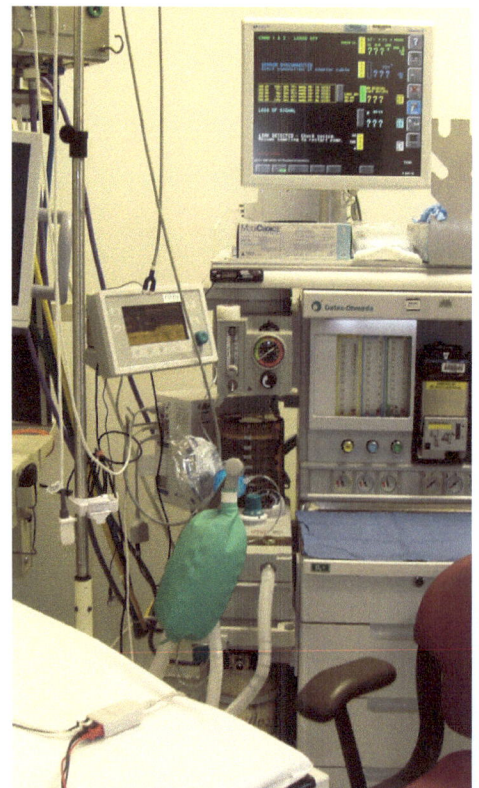

Liver Transplant Liver Transplant Set-Up

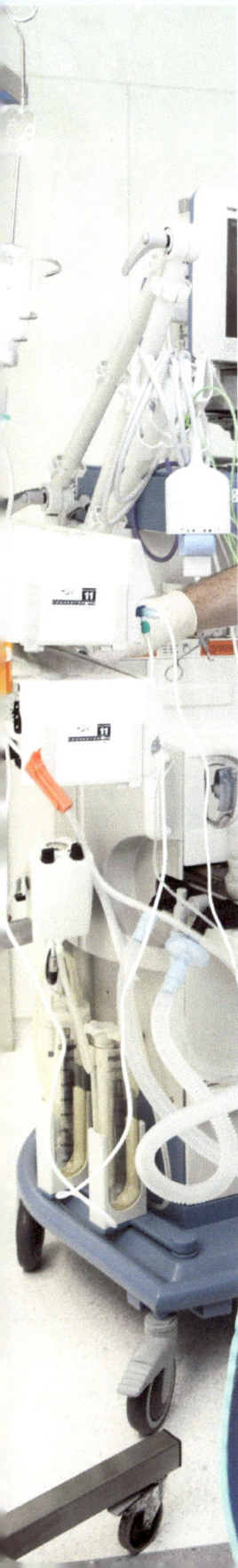

1. Call secretary and verify the time and location of the liver transplant.

2. Ask secretary to print patient labels.

3. Get SvO2 cable (if needed)

4. Verify TEGS are QC'd

5. Verify that the liver transplant room has the following:

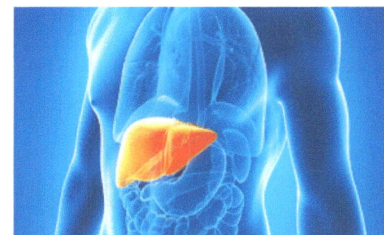

  a. BH machine x2, UBBH, LBBH

  b. H₂O-blanket machine

  c. Vigilance monitor

  d. 4 pressure modules, art-line and CVP modules   connected to vigilance

  e. Headboard (often found in liver prep room)

  f. ACD x 2

  g. Programmable infusion pumps x 3

  h. BIS monitor

  i. Site-rite

  j. Prep liver cart

6. Set up cell-saver (including paperwork).

Use ACD only; do NOT use heparin. Set up double reservoir, only if requested.

7. Set up a Level One (dry) for backup.

8. Get wire cart from workroom/stock room and collect the following:

  a. Anything missing from liver transplant room

  b. ABG reqs. X 10, lab requires. X 20, 514s x 10

  c. BIS sensors x 2

  d. Extra towels

  e. 1-liter bags of normal saline (sodium chloride) x 6

  f. Tx1 and Tx3 (you are responsible for flushing transducers)

  g. Swan (PA) catheter

  h. 9 Fr. introducer kit x 2

  i. RIC

  j. Clipboards x 3

9. From the equipment room, retrieve:

  a. Thermacor or Belmont (disposables in stock room)

  b. Liver cart (verify it is properly stocked)

  c. Blood gas machine 10. Set up and prime Thermacor or Belmont

11. Check for patient labels and SVO2 cable

12. Verify level 1 TEG controls are in. If not, repeat; if so, run level 2 controls

13. Set up the room:

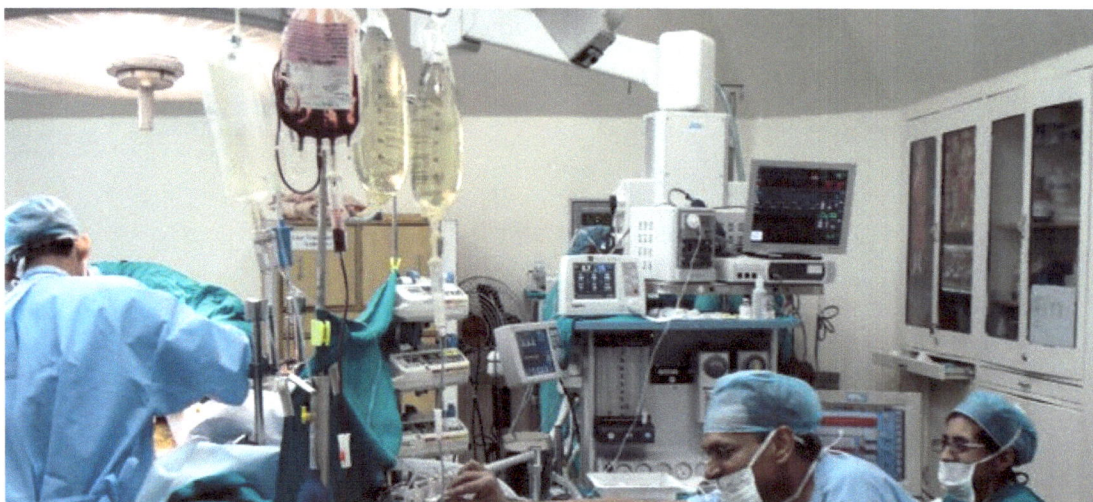

  a. Put cell-saver in the hallway

  b. Put Level One in the hallway

  c. Place Thermacor and one BH machine with UBBH to the left of the bed and plug in.

  d. Place second Bair Hugger machine under the foot of the bed. Place LBBH at the foot of bed.

  e. Replace all LR in anesthesia cart with normal saline (sodium chloride).

  f. Place 9 Fr. introducers, RIC and art-line caddie on liver prep cart. Put cart next to anesthesia cart.

  g. Put headboard on the bed and prep with towels.

  h. Place transducers on the headboard (Tx3 on the right, Tx1 on the left) and zero.

  i. Tape Swan to the square table. j. Get patient labels and do paperwork.

  j.i. Stamp stickers (40), ABG/lactate reqs. X 10, Lab reqs. x 10, 514's x 5, RIS sheet, cell-saver sheet, and ABG result sheet (ABG/lactate reqs., ABG result sheet, and RIS sheet should be found on the side of the liver cart).

  j.ii. Tape 514 forms on the wall behind anesthesia cart. Label two RBCs, two FFP, and one Cryo/platelets.

  j.iii. Place RIS and ABG result sheets on a clipboard and hang from RIS (aka Rapid Infusion System = Thermacor/Belmont). j.iv. Place stickers, ABG reqs., and lab reqs. on the liver cart.

k. Prepare for blood tests.

   k.i. Open and set aside 10-ml syringes, blood gas syringes, and a 20-ml syringe.

   k.ii. Set aside unsterile 3x3 sponges and needles.

   k.iii. Label 5 lavender tops, 5 blue tops, and 1 red top tube and place in the rack.

14. When the patient arrives in pre-an. a. Get information on the patient for vigilance (height, weight, hematocrit). b. Ask the anesthesia provider how much blood to order (standard amount is 20 units RBCs, and 10 units FFP). c. Call blood bank and verify they are thawing FFP and tell them how much blood is to be put in a cooler d. Hook up SVO2 cable, enter information and calibrate.

15. Verify that the level 2 TEG controls have come in; rerun if necessary. Return TEG levers to load and set up for patient testing. Enter patient data.

Donor Room Set-Up

- Tx2
- Level One
- BPx3 BH machine x 2,
- UBBH, LBBH
- H2O Blanket under gel pad, machine
- Cell-saver (possible double reservoir) ACD only

Donor liver immediately after donation

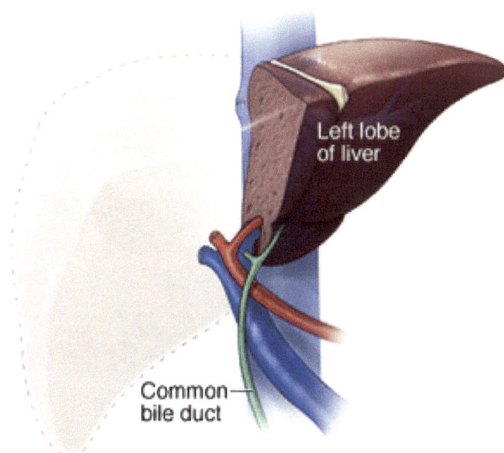

Donor liver two months after donation

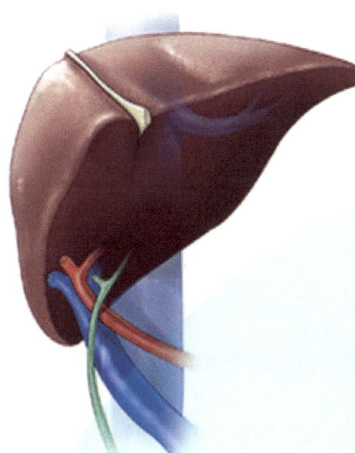

Left lobe of liver

Common bile duct

Pediatric Set Ups TPANG

- Level 1
- No RIS or CS
- Tx2 and Tx1
- Pediatric tubes
- Draw little amounts of blood
- Peds full access BH

When the Patient is in the Room

1. Assist with patient prep. (This may include helping to intubate, place lines,   oat the swan, etc.)

2. When the art-line is in the patient, draw first set of labs.

a. Run blood gas. SAVE BLOOD and send up to the lab with coags for baseline lactate.

b. Send coags. Include hematocrit, platelet, PT, PTT, fibrinogen, and magnesium (red, blue and lavender tubes). Be sure to label blood tubes.

c. Run a TEG (kaolin only). 3. When IV lines are in, call to verify that blood is ready. Get blood cooler from the blood bank and have it checked.

4. Bring in cell-saver when requested.

5. Wash RBCs if necessary.

a. Get a Y-set from the perfusion rack in center core 2 (Y-type blood set may be used if Y-set is not available) and hook it up to the suction reservoir of the cell-saver.

b. Spike the RBC units. Save the transfusion stickers and label them as washed to put on 514s

c. When the blood is in the reservoir, wash the blood following the usual cell-saver procedure. Do not   ll out paperwork.

d. They usually ask for 5 units to be washed. Split the blood up in bags (at least two) to store the blood in and place in cooler if not used immediately. Record as washed units when given to the patient

_____

e. When completed, turn off the cell-saver to reset the numbers.

f. When they start getting a significant blood loss, discontinue washing RBC units or use another cell-saver for the patient.

During the Case

1. Clean Site-Rite and return to cardiac rooms.

2. Every half hour, draw up a partial set of blood labs and run a blood gas.

3. Every hour, withdraw a full blood set.

   a. Run a blood gas. SAVE BLOOD and send to lab coags for lactate (check LACTATE ONLY on ABG/lactate req.).

   b. Send coags. Include hematocrit, platelet, PT, PTT (blue and lavender tubes).

   c. Run a normal TEG.

4. Record blood work results as they come in. Call for results if not received promptly.

5. Draw up and run lab work as requested.

6. Fill Thermacor with blood products and crystalloid as requested.
Do NOT throw out used bags; set them aside in pink buckets.

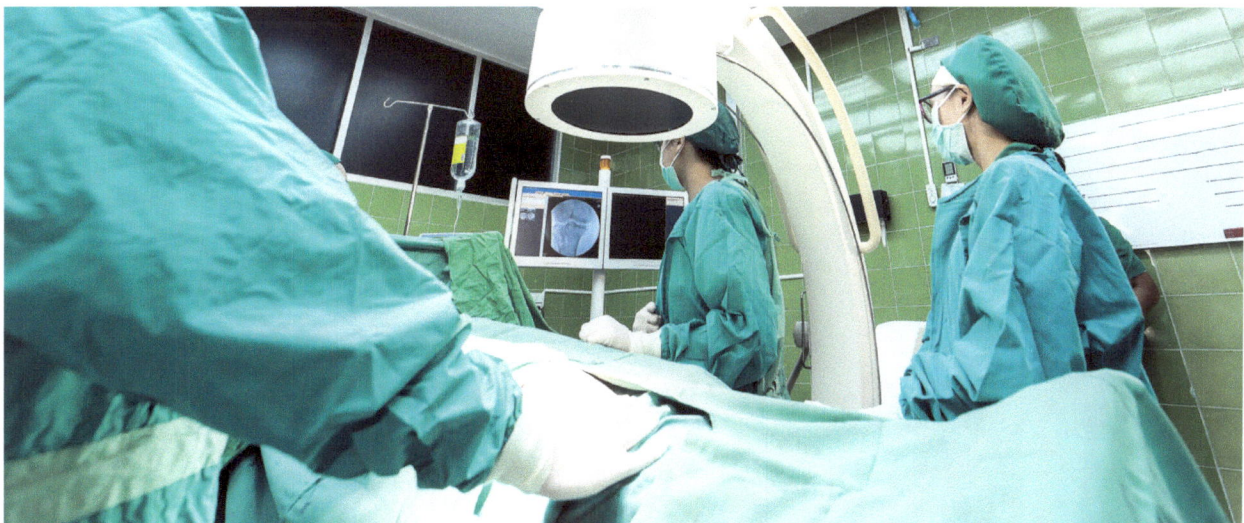

7. Fill out RIS sheet

  a. Record fluid put in Thermacor and blood products used.

  b. Circle blood products not put in Thermacor but given directly to the patient through IV.

  c. Write "washed" next to units if they have been washed.

  d. Place blood product labels on 514 sheets.

8. Run cell-saver. (This includes filling out the cell-saver sheet. It is a good idea to check reservoir levels every time you draw a blood gas.)

9. Assist clinicians as needed.

Before Reperfusion

Observe sterile technique at all times.

1. Set up TEG for Amicar (aminocaproic acid) and Protamine (protamine sulfate) samples.

  a. In specimen cups, mix up Amicar and Protamine samples.

    a.i. Amicar (Aminocaproic Acid): Mix 3.0ml aminocaproic acid in 50ml normal saline.

    a.ii. Protamine (Protamine Sulfate): Mix 3.6ml Protamine in 50ml normal saline.

  b. Set up TEG sample cups for three samples: normal, Amicar, and Protamine (when inputting data, be sure to choose correct sample type).

2. Set up syringes, blood tubes (including red) and paperwork for blood draws and testing at reperfusion.

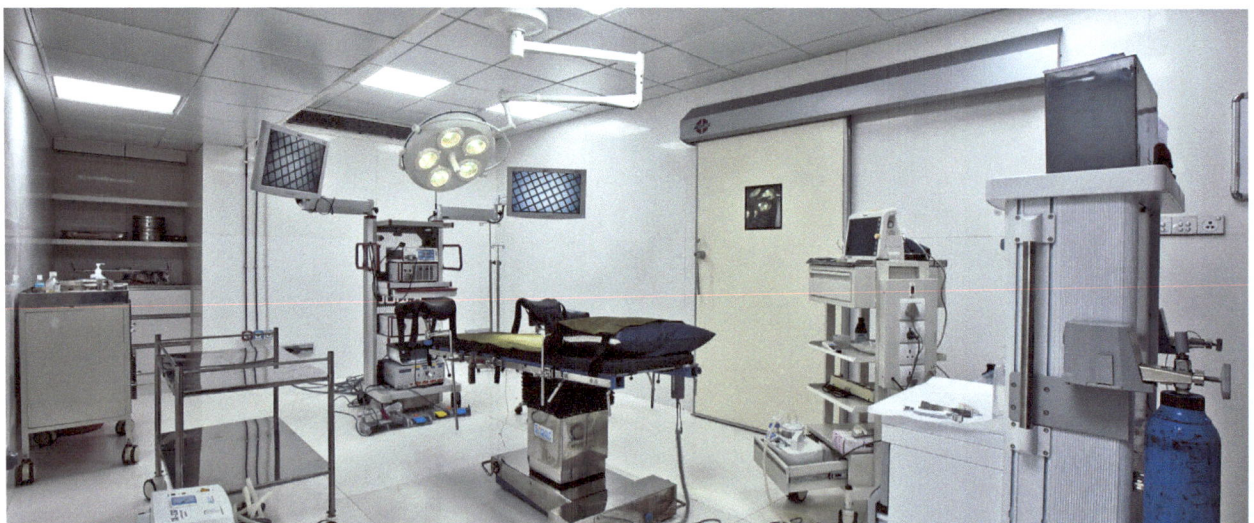

Reperfusion

1. 30 seconds after reperfusion, draw a blood gas. SAVE BLOOD and send a sample to the lab with coags for lactate (check LACTATE ONLY on ABG/lactate req.).

2. 5 minutes after reperfusion, draw a full set.

   a. Run blood gas. SAVE THE BLOOD sample and send it up to the lab with coags for lactate (check LACTATE ONLY on ABG/lactate req.).

   b. Send coags. Include hematocrit, platelet, PT, PTT, fibrinogen, and magnesium (red, blue, and lavender tubes). Be sure to label blood tubes.

   c. Run TEG samples (normal, Amicar (Aminocaproic Acid) and Protamine (Protamine Sulfate)). For Amicar and Protamine, use the QC pipettes to put 20uL of the drug in the cup, and then add 340 uL of blood. All samples should be kaolin activated.

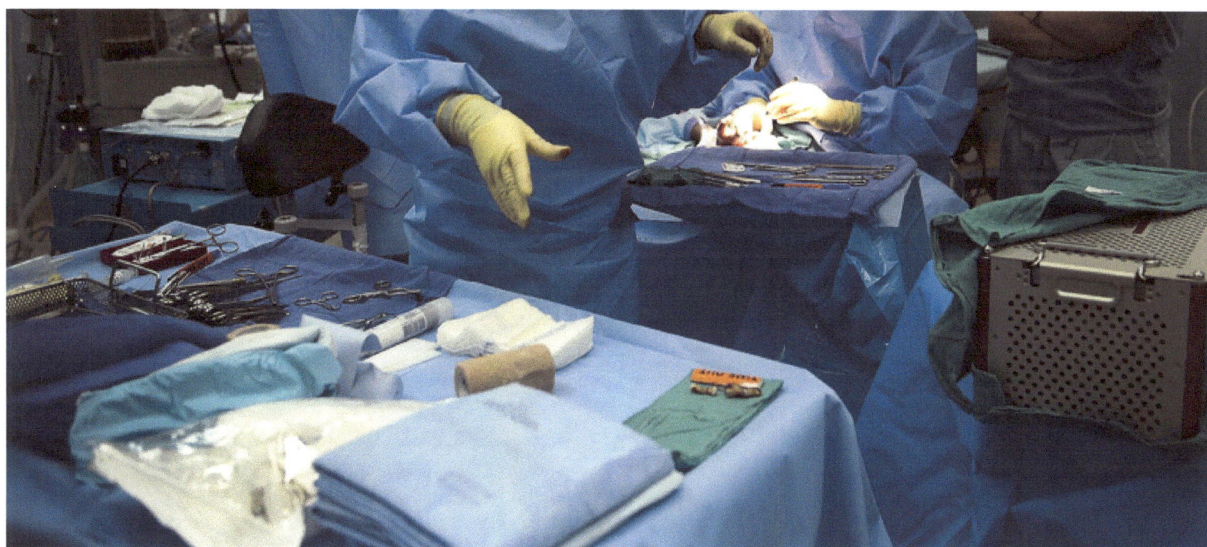

After Reperfusion

1. Continue with procedures as listed above under "During the Case."

2. Begin restocking and cleaning room, as time permits.

End of Case

1. Set up ICU bed for transport.

2. Get travel cooler for transport.

    a. Ask anesthesia provider how many RBCs and FFPs they want in the travel cooler.

    b. Call blood bank and inform them you are about to come up for the travel cooler for the liver transplant.

    c. Get wire cart and bring liver cooler up to the blood bank (ground floor by red elevators).

    d. Bring travel cooler down and put on the bed.

3. Verify the blood product numbers on the RIS sheet match up with stickers on 514 sheets. If not, recount bags and/or search for missing stickers/bags. Give numbers to the clinician.

4. Complete ABG result sheet (call lab if needed for missing results).

5. Give clinician RIS sheet, ABG result sheet, and 514s.

6. Help with transferring patient to bed and/or transporting the patient to the unit if needed.

7. Turn over the room.

8. Clean cell-saver and rapid infuser system and return to workroom.

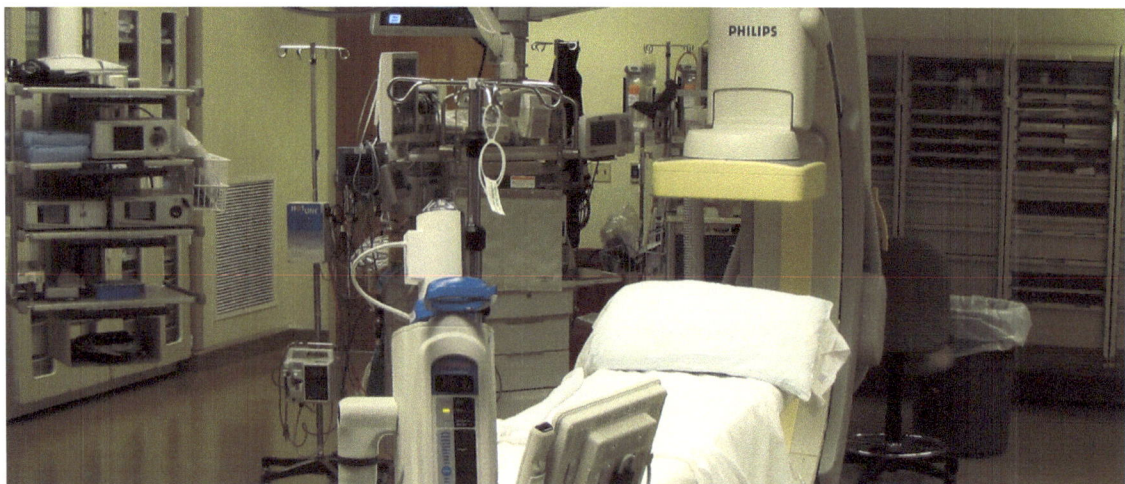

Cardiac
Cardiac Room Setup Checklist

- 4 Programmable infusion pumps
- Machine with circuit on it
- Bis-monitor with strip and alcohol swabs taped on top
- Ranger warmer
- Bair hugger

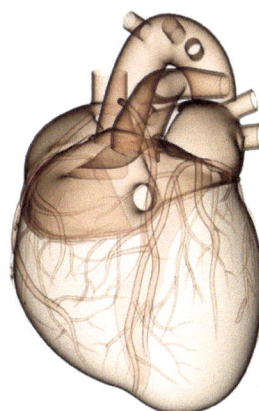

**ALL ON
IV POLE**

- Clean TEE probe
- TEE machine with twill tape and black TEE holder
- Vigilance monitor with CCO and SvO2 cables
- Ultrasound of some variety with ultrasound covers and gel
- Cardiac trauma cart with 3 extra programmable infusion pumps
- Level 1(Dry Setup)
- 3-tiered cart (top with 9Fr 10cm introducer, sterile gloves, gown and Biopatch)
- EKG leads on bed (green and white leads to the right; red, brown, and black to the left)
- Triple transducer with pressure bag hanging on right side of bed
- Swan (PA) catheter taped to table with Durapore tape
- Cardiac Anesthesia Technical Support Procedures

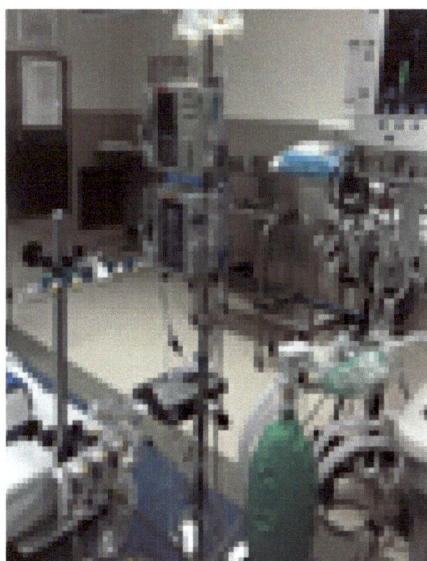

Transesophageal Echocardiogram

- **(TEE) Machine**

- Always kept in heart rooms. The small portable TEE machine/ultrasound should always be kept plugged in. The extra TEE probe is kept in the room where the probes are cleaned.

- Clear the top of all extra items. The only items that should be on top of this machine are umbilical tape, a pair of scissors, aquasonic gel, heart, and latex-free gloves (S,M,L).

- The TEE probe is very expensive and more fragile than it looks. Please keep it in the plexiglass tubes whenever possible. Except for cleaning, inspection, and insertion, the TEE probe should be stored in one of these plexiglass tubes.

- Provide the multi-plane probes for all adult cardiac rooms running. If a peds case is scheduled, peds cardiology will bring down their own probe and machine, so store our probes in the office by Room 4 behind the door.

- Clean probes are now placed in a clean plastic sheath and inside a protective tube taped and marked "clean" and placed on the rack mounted on the wall by the anesthesia cart in the rooms.

- Turn the machine on. Make sure an image comes up on the screen. If any error messages come up, write the message down exactly and relay it to the supervisor.

- Enter patient's name, medical record #, age, anesthesia attending's initials, surgeon's name, indication for surgery, and procedure.

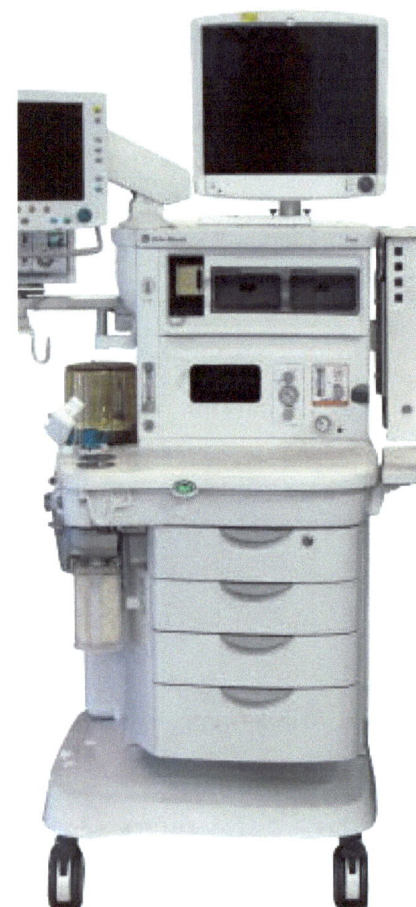

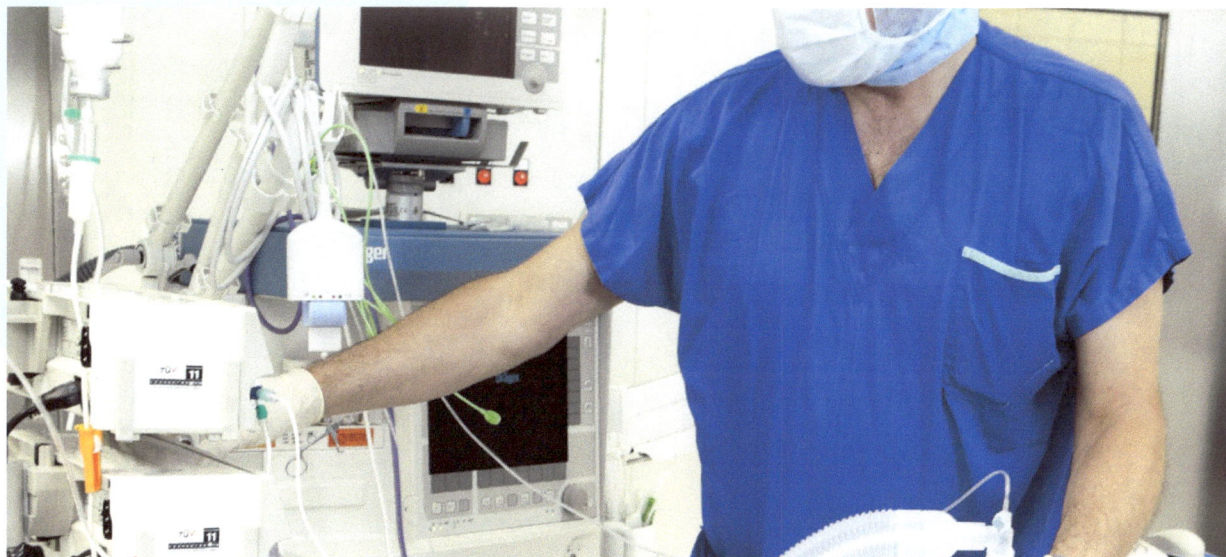

- Make sure the probe is clean. Crust or stains should be removed from the TEE probe prior to disinfection. If there are any residuals on the probe after it has been disinfected, these should be removed and the probe disinfected again.

- Finally, make sure that the black spiral cable is plugged into the DCA port on the left-hand side of the TEE machine and the other end plugged into the monitor boom.

- Ensure that the ethernet cable is plugged into the back of the TEE machine and the other end is plugged into the monitor boom.

- Ensure the video coaxial cable is plugged into the back of the machine inside the back cabinet door, and the coaxial cable is plugged into the video color output spot, and make sure the other end is plugged into the aux 1 port on the monitor boom.

- Last, make sure there is a black spiral cable plugged into the front of the Phillips patient monitor on top of the gas machine in the port marked ECG and that the other end is plugged into the port on the boom.

Cardiac Kit Cart

Adults: Place a blue towel on the top shelf, along with a 9Fr kit, a sterile gown, and sterile gloves, size 7 ½. The second shelf should have (from left to right) at least (2) 9Fr introducer kits, and at least (2) 9Fr MAC introducer kits. All extra items must be removed from this cart and put away in the workroom.

For pediatric patients: Cook central venous catheter trays are used (sizes vary). The resident will acquire or ask a tech to bring this.

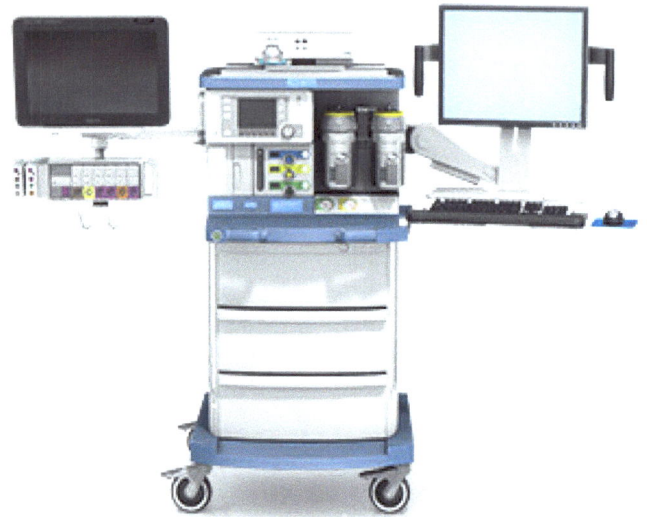

Trauma Cart

Each pump room has its own trauma cart. Check this cart to make sure nothing is missing. The cart has a metal basket hanging on the right side. In it belongs autologous blood collection kits and BIS monitor sensors. One 500ml pressure bag and one 1000ml pressure bag must be hanging from this cart. If there is more than one of each, remove the extras and take back to the workroom. Across the top of the trauma cart, left to right, should be the large drug labels, programmable infusion pumps (x2-3), and pink buckets (x2).

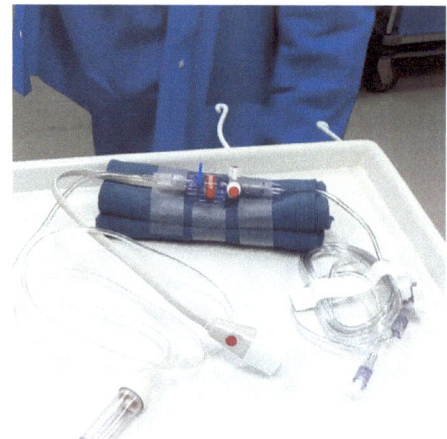

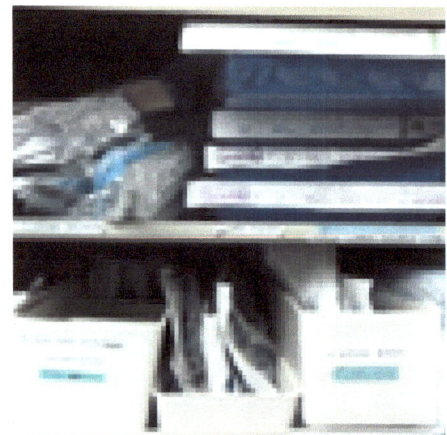

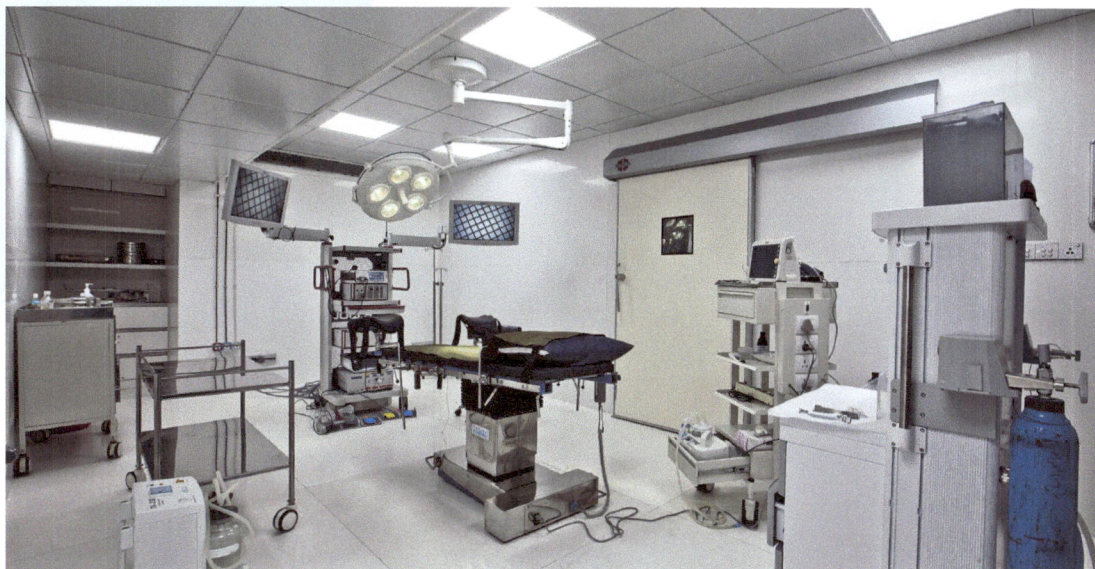

Site-Rite (Ultrasound)

Make sure each pump room has a site-rite with charged batteries (or a plug). Make sure the Site-Rite is clean. The basket attached to the Site-Rite must have plenty of Site-Rite sheaths in it and a bottle of aquasonic gel.

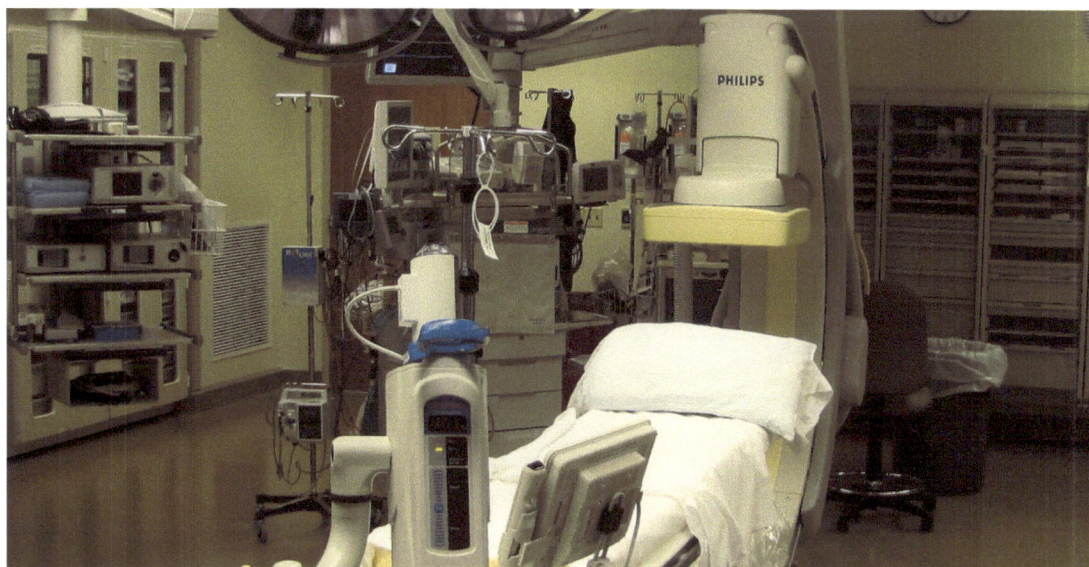

Anesthesia Machine

Anesthesia providers typically set up the following:

   A) On top of the machine, place a Mac 3 blade with a handle you have tested

   B) A Miller-2 blade with a tested handle

   C) 7.5 and 8.0 ET tube left closed in package

   D) A stylet and a 10-ml syringe

   E) 2 sponges

   F) A tongue blade, 90, oral airway (leave others in cart)

   G) A role of Transpore and a role of Durapore tape ANESTHESIA TECHNICIAN SURVIVAL

If using the smaller packaged Swan-ganz, tape the cardiac output temp probe to the bag you have prepped (#4). Make sure CCO and regular CO cables and Swan are available. Do not open Swan unless requested. If using combo Swan, bag #4 is not needed. The SVO2 cable will be needed. Please note that the SVO2 cable will go back to the unit with the patient.

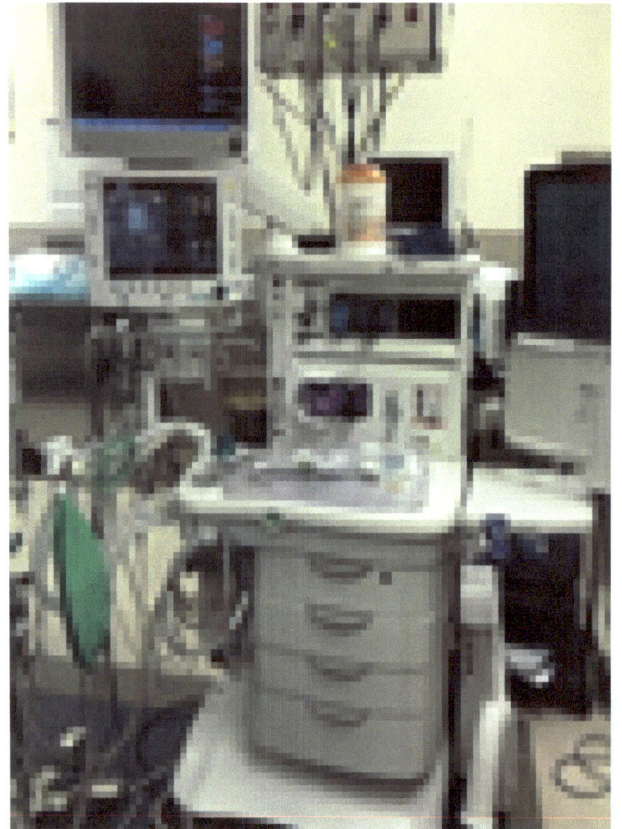

IV Lines

These are set up for potential or real emergency cases or when an anesthesia provider does not have a resident to do it for them. They must be available at all times. Beware of expiration times and dates. Write time and date and your initials when you prepare them.

#1 & #2: 2 sets (one on left and one on the right) of 1000 ml LR macro drip spike plus 1 Walrus set.

#3 on the right, 1000 ml NS spiked with micro drip, followed by 5 stopcocks.

As needed, set up by resident: 1000 ml NS spiked with Y blood set to Ranger followed by 1 Walrus set.

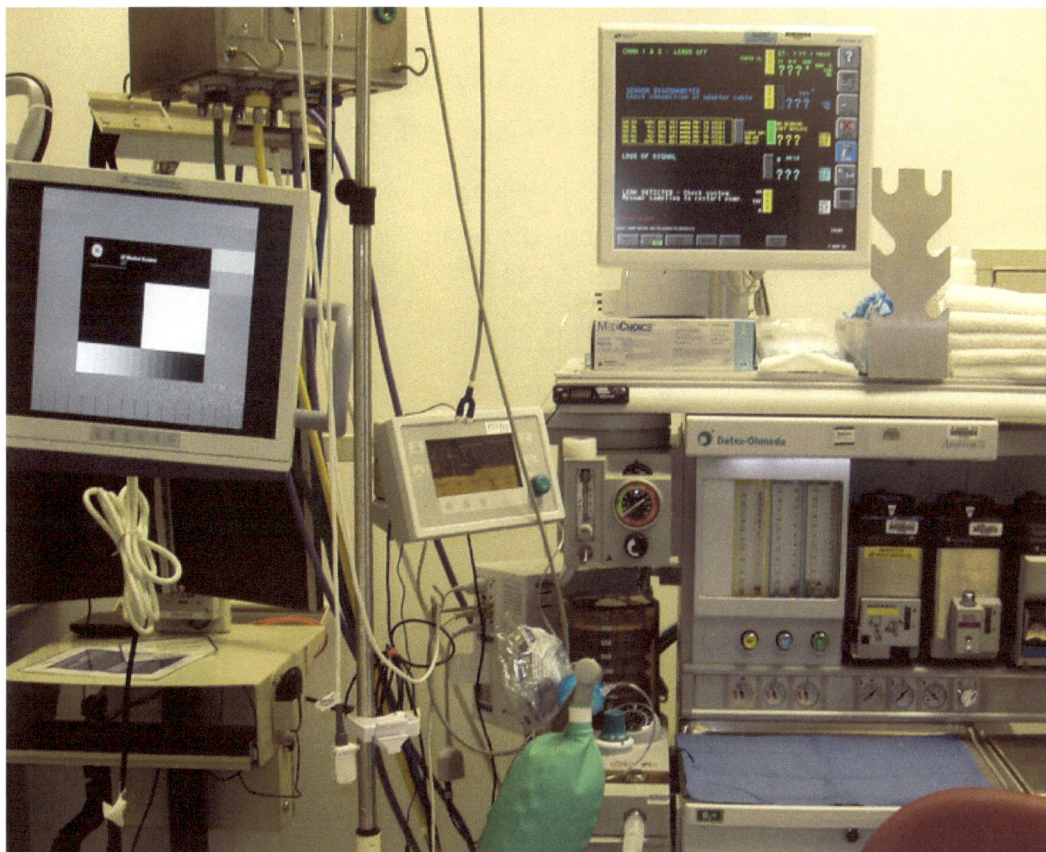

Provide Transducer: Adult

Attach Tx3 to transduced ped-pole (or bed pole) as opposed to IV poles. Make sure bag is hung on one of the right-side bedrails as opposed to directly on the pole itself. Hook the transducer up to the modules and zero. Make sure zero holds and pressure bag is inflated enough (300). Make sure bag has not expired. Keep transducer cables NEATLY wrapped up, so they do not drag on the floor or get in the way, only if the short transducer cables are not available.

Continuous Cardiac Output (CCO) Swan Setup:

In most adult cases, the CCO Swan must be hooked up prior to the patient entering the room.

The CCO Swan needs to be removed from its sterile bag and placed on a prep table (provided by the cardiac nurses) on the right side of the OR bed. Tape the plastic Swan container to the prep table using the transport tape.

Move the small plastic cover on the CCO Swan package (the one covering the blue, yellow and white ports and small syringe).

Remove the small syringe.

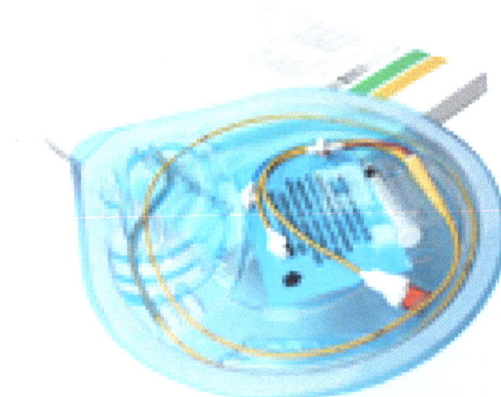

Draw the syringe back to the 1 and ½ ml mark and connect it to the red line on the CCO Swan.

The blue line (CVP) and yellow (PA distal) get connected to their respective transducer lines and stop-cocks turned to 45 degrees so that uid won't exit the tubes by gravity.

The white (VIP) should also be connected to the micro-drip I.V. with the stopcock manifold.
Calibrate the SV02 cable as well.

OR Bed and Monitors

- Make sure a **water blanket** is on the bed under a full body gel pad and is attached to the water blanket machine.

- Make sure the clamps are open.

- Turn on the water machine to make sure it is working.
- Fill when necessary.

- Lay out **ECG leads and place electrodes** on them. White and green on patient's right side; black, red, and brown on the left. Tuck under the warming blanket.

- **Pulse ox.** The clip is hung on patient's left side. Test to make sure it is working.

- NBP cuff is tucked under the mattress at patient's head.

- **BIS:** Make sure a BIS monitor is attached to the Ranger IV pole, the cables are wrapped neatly, and a BIS sensor is set on top. Check power.

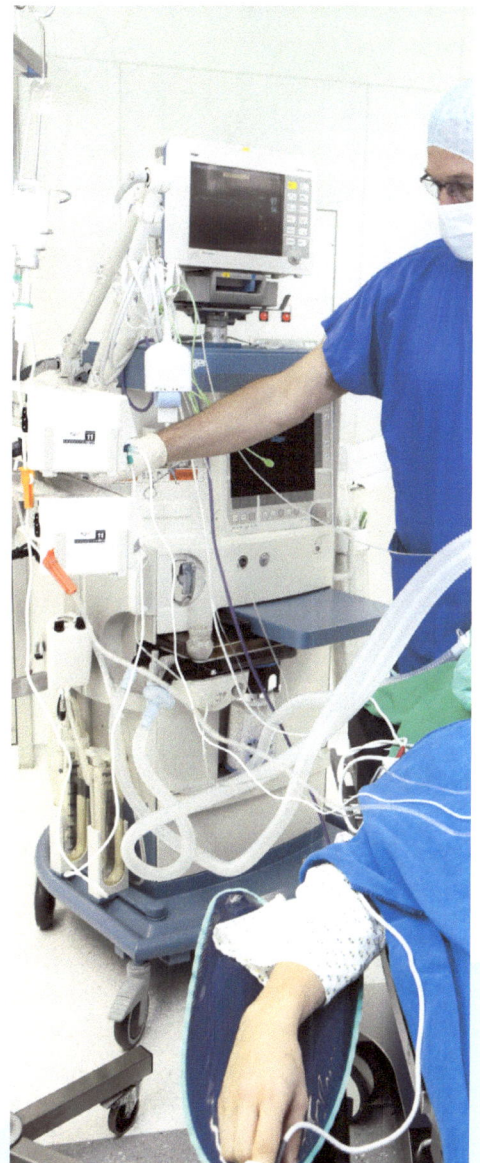

• Rectal probe: Keep 2x stored in the **middle drawer of gas machine.**

Extra items to store in 2nd drawer of the gas machine:

- 1 x pulse ox cable and clip

- 2 x each adult disposable pulse ox varieties (green and blue packages)

- 2 x disposal skin temperature sensors

- 1 x ECG cable and leads

- The cardiac output temperature probe cable if it is not in use

Assisting the Cardiac Anesthesia Provider

Help bring the patient into OR and transfer to OR bed. Help put monitors on the patient.

Assist intubation.

- Apply cricoid pressure when requested.
- Hand-off ET tube and remove stylet when requested.
- Hold tube in place until taped.
- Monitor patient's blood pressure at all times and especially after anesthesiologist puts on sterile gloves. Connect IV line to the side port of the 9Fr catheter when it is in place. (Drip # 1) Hand Swan catheter to anesthesiologist using sterile technique.

Help float Swan.

- Start with the balloon down.
- Do as requested and announce what you have done as you do it, saying, "Balloon is up" or, "Balloon is down."
- Be responsive because balloon must be down when the Swan is pulled back.

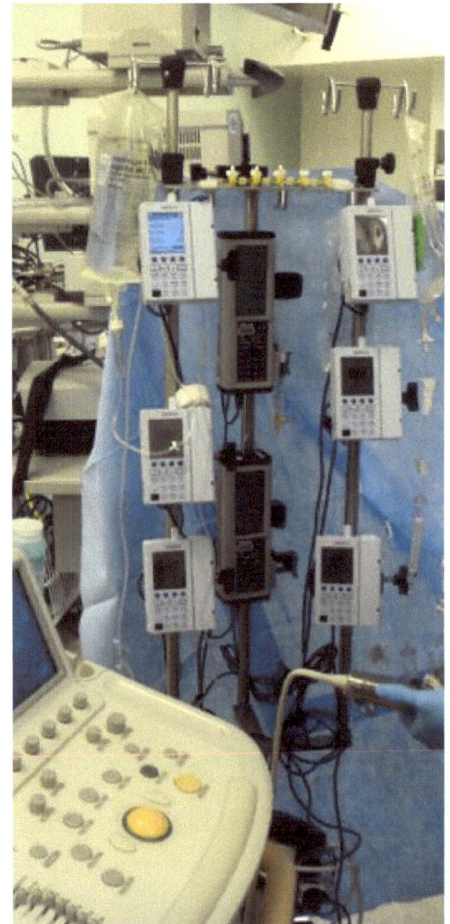

Other Items That Belong in Cardiac Rooms at All Times:

  a) Level-1 machine set up "dry."

  b) Bair hugger machine with both upper and lower blankets available. Any items borrowed from the cardiac rooms must be returned/replaced ASAP.

When assisting the cardiac anesthesia provider so that the resident can get the next case interviewed and place vascular lines in pre-an area:

At the direction of the cardiac anesthesia attending, the cardiac anesthesia technician should be available to assist continuously for approximately 20 – 30 minutes in the last hour of the case. This will greatly expedite turnover by allowing the resident to see and to prepare the next patient for their anesthesia and surgery

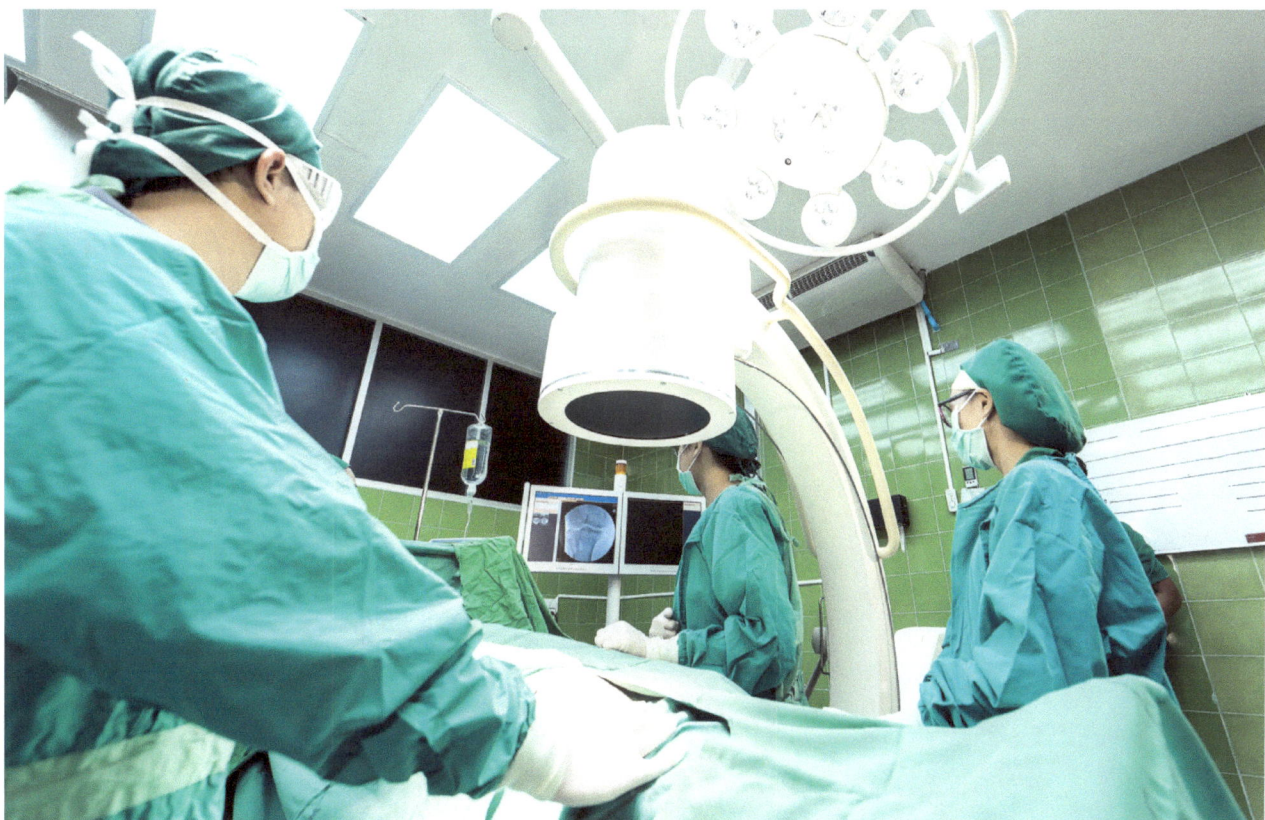

Swan Calibration and Vigilance Monitor Setup

- After setting up the Swan, turn on the vigilance CCO monitor, connect the SV02 cable (Grey) and the CCO cable (white) to the monitor, then the other ends to the Swan.

- On the right-hand side of the CCO screen, press the button that says, "Patient Data." The screen will then change.

- Now at the bottom of the screen, press the button that says, "New Patient." It will ask you if you want to clear patient data profiles; press "yes."

- If there is a button at the bottom of the screen that says "Ht/Wt/BSA," press it. If not, go to the right side of the screen and press "EDIT."

- Press "CURSOR" until the highlighted block on the screen is on height (enter the patient's height), then hit the "cursor" button until it highlights weight (enter weight), then press "return" and then "Home."

- On the main screen at the bottom, press the button "SV02."

- Press "invitro."

- Press on the right side of the button that says "Cal." Wait 20 sec. for the screen to say "Invitro calibration O.K."

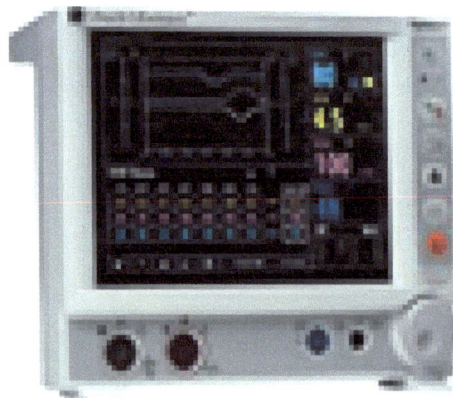

- You are done.

Tee Setup

Check to make sure all the connections from the TEE machine are connected properly

Power up the machine. The power button is located below the screen on the left-hand side.

After the machine is powered up and the screen is fully booted, press the "Begin End" button located on the far upper left-hand corner of the control board (keyboard)

After pressing "Begin End," the patient information screen will come up.

Enter in all the information (first and last name, medical record number, etc.).

After all the information is entered, press the "Patient Data" button located on the right-hand side of the roller mouse. • Press the title cursor button and type in the name of the procedure.
\
Press the title cursor again.

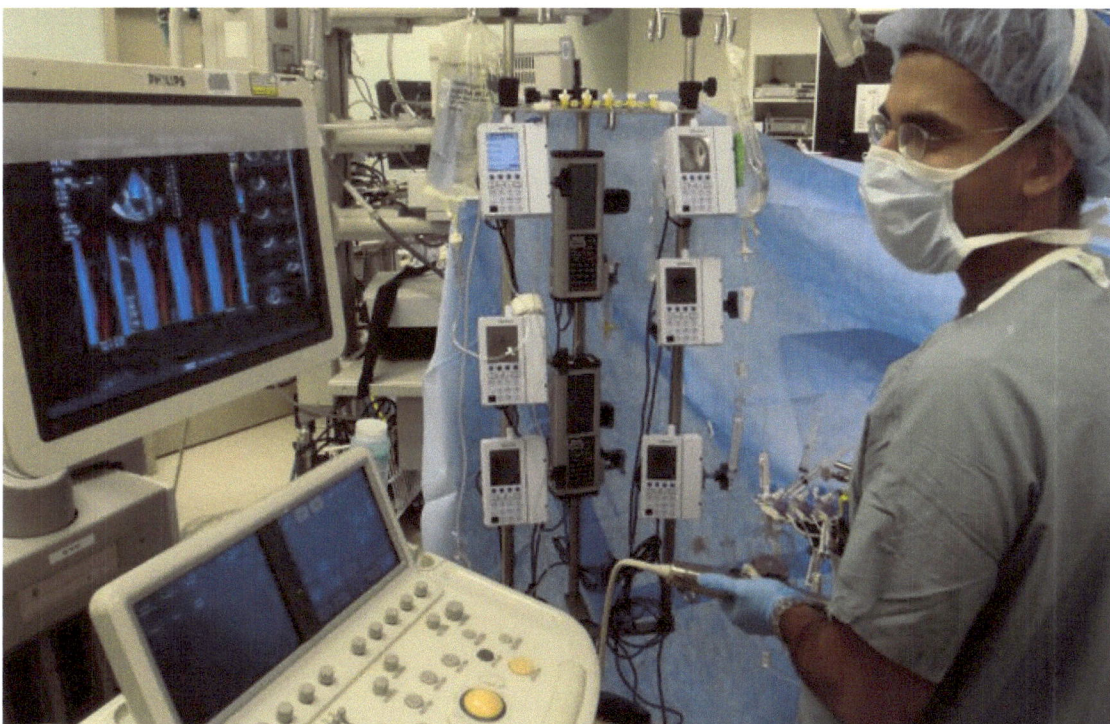

SPECIALIZED SETUPS BY CASE

1) Aortic Reconstruction (Abdominal Aortic Aneurysm, Aorto-bifem bypass, etc

   A) Arterial Line

   B) CVP or swan-Ganz catheter

   C) Fluid Warmer (Hotline or Ranger)

   D) Warming Blanket E) Epidural vs intrathecal tray

2) Carotid Endarterectomy A) Arterial Line

3) Thoracotomy/Tharaco-abdominal

   A) Arterial Line

   B) Fluid Warmer

   C) Warming Blanket

   D) Epidural vs Intrathecal tray

   E) Double-lumen Endobronchial Tube

   F) Fiberoptic Airway Cart

4) Thoracoscopy

A) Double-lumen Endobronchial Tube B) Fiberoptic Airway Cart C) Possible Arterial line

5) Major Intra-Abdominal (Cystectomy, Nephrectomy, GYN Exploratory/ Omentectomy/Para-aortic Lymph Nodes)

   A) Fluid Warmer

   B) Warming Blanket

   C) Possible invasive lines (Arterial Line, CVP, Swan)

   D) Epidural vs Intrathecal Tray

6) Major Spine

   A) Warming Blanket

   B) Fluid Warmer

   C) Possible Arterial Line

   D) Possible second IV

7) Craniotomy

    A) Arterial Line

    B) Warming Blanket

    C) Fluid Warmer

THE FUTURE

Noninvasive monitoring is the future, but some will say it is the now.

There are a few companies that have come up with the technology to perform noninvasive monitoring; This technology has some anesthesia technicians paying very close attention.

Edwards Lifescience's Clearsight system is one of them:

The ClearSight System

A simple, noninvasive approach to monitoring key hemodynamic parameters.

- Stroke Volume (SV)
- Stroke Volume Variation (SVV)
- Cardiac Output (CO)
- Systemic Vascular Resistance (SVR)
- Continuous Blood Pressure (cBP)

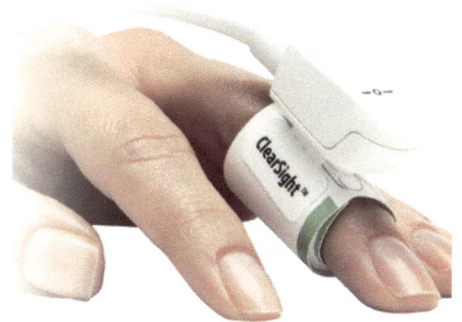

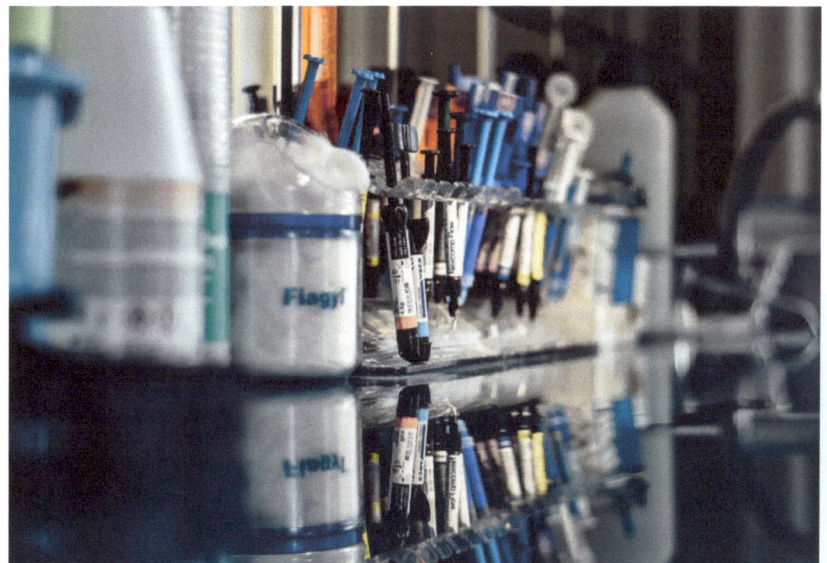

CLEARSIGHT SYSTEM

Noninvasive simplicity. Next-generation clarity.

The noninvasive ClearSight system provides valuable hemodynamic insight to an expanded patient population, for making more informed decisions about volume administration in moderate to high-risk surgery.

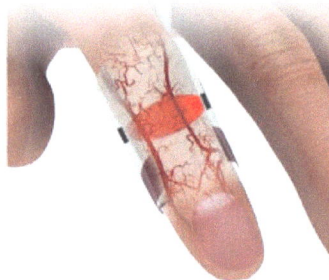

- **ClearSight System Technology**
  The technology is based on two methods: the volume clamp method to continuously measure Blood Pressure and the Physiocal method for initial and frequent calibration. The essence of the volume clamp method involves clamping the artery to a constant volume by dynamically providing equal pressure on either side of the arterial wall. The volume is measured by a photo-plethysmograph built into the cuff.

Delivering clarity in every moment.

The ClearSight system quickly connects to the patient by wrapping an inflatable cuff around the finger. The simplicity of the ClearSight system gives you noninvasive access to automatic, up-to-the-minute hemodynamic information for a broader patient population, including elderly or obese patients in whom an arterial catheter would not typically be placed. Thus, enabling you to make more informed decisions regarding volume administration.

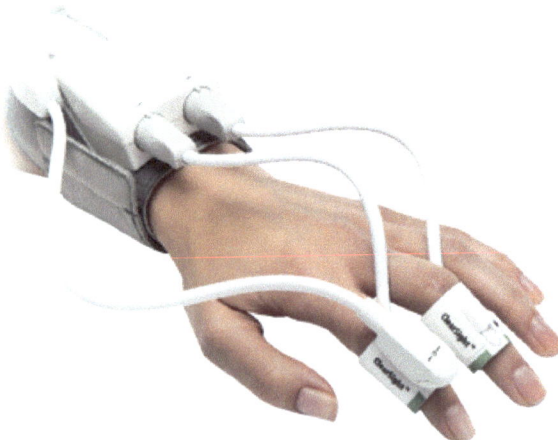

- **ClearSight Finger Cuff**
  The ClearSight finger cuff provides up to 72 hours of valuable hemodynamic insight. Continuous monitoring on one finger is limited to 8 hours. However, uninterrupted monitoring over 8 hours is possible using two cuffs on two fingers.

A simple, noninvasive approach to monitoring key hemodynamic parameters.

Dynamic and flow-based parameters such as SV and SVV, provided by the ClearSight system may be used in perioperative goal-directed therapy (PGDT) protocols and are key to optimal volume administration for patients at risk of developing complications.

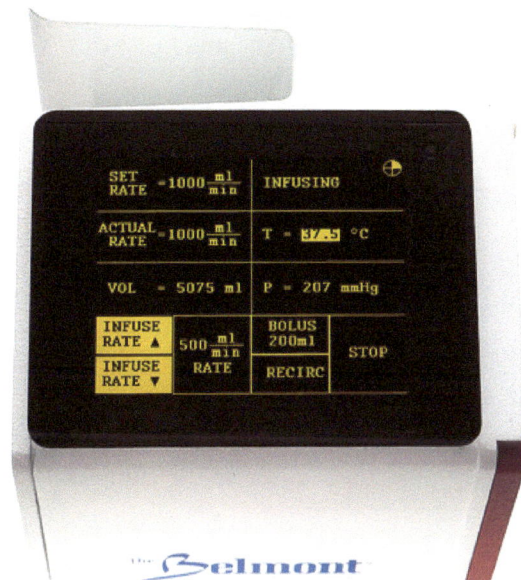

Another is Cheetah Medical's Unique cheetah sensor technology:

100% noninvasive hemodynamic monitoring

CHEETAH Sensors are 100% noninvasive, easy to apply and can be placed on the front or back of the patient as necessitated by the patient's position, clinical condition or procedure requirements.

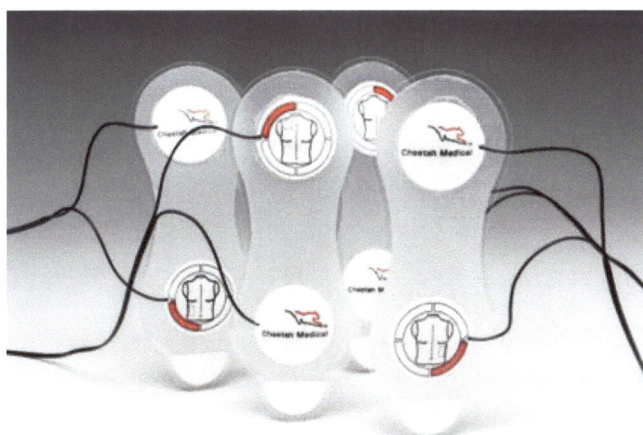

Our Sensors consist of a double-electrode configuration with two simultaneous functions. The first function is to deliver the continuous low-voltage alternating electrical current supplied by the Cheetah monitor. The second function is to continuously receive the signal emanating from the patient.

These signals are then analyzed by the **CHEETAH NICOM™** or **STARLING™ SV** monitors to determine stroke volume (SV), heart rate, cardiac output (CO), and other hemodynamic information.

Key Features

- 100% noninasive
- Easy to apply by either a nurse, physician or technician
- Non-latex
- Can be used for up to 48 hours
- Flexible sensor location: can be applied to the front or back of a patient
- Phthalates-free

100% NONINVASIVE VOLUME MANAGEMENT TO GUIDE CLINICAL DECISION-MAKING

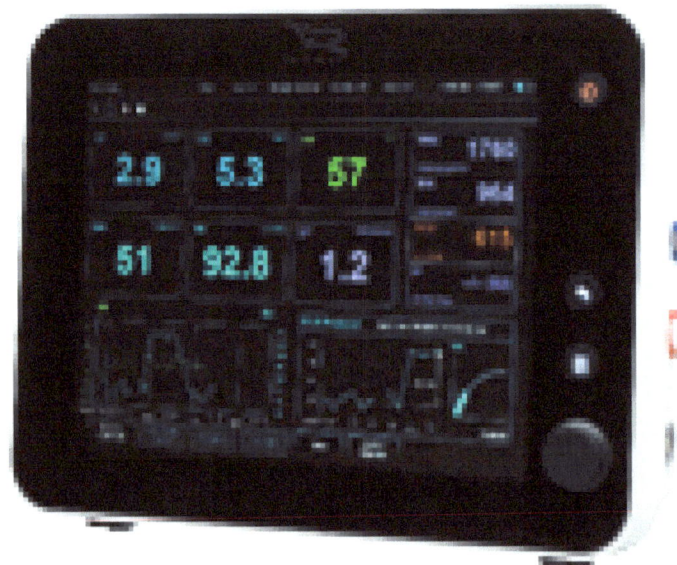

Our Sensors consist of a double-electrode configuration with two simultaneous functions. The first function is to deliver the continuous low-voltage alternating electrical current supplied by the Cheetah monitor. The second function is to continuously receive the signal emanating from the patient.

These signals are then analyzed by the **CHEETAH NICOM™** or **STARLING™ SV** monitors to determine stroke volume (SV), heart rate, cardiac output (CO), and other hemodynamic information.

Key Features

- 100% noninasive
- Easy to apply by either a nurse, physician or technician
- Non-latex
- Can be used for up to 48 hours
- Flexible sensor location: can be applied to the front or back of a patient
- Phthalates-free

100% NONINVASIVE VOLUME MANAGEMENT TO GUIDE CLINICAL DECISION-MAKING

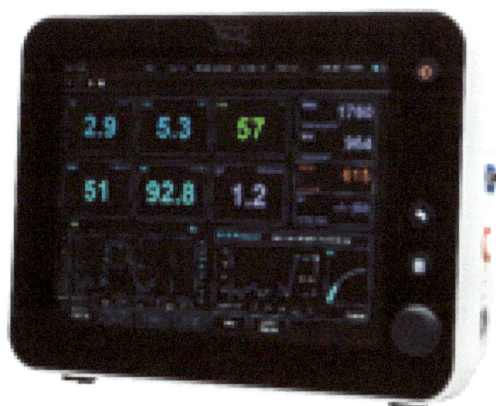

The Cheetah Starling™ SV hemodynamic monitoring system provides the ability to obtain 100% noninvasive dynamic assessments of uid responsiveness to guide volume management.

The Starling™ SV system is designed to give clinicians the full hemodynamic picture of their patient.

Because the device measures centrally, it provides accurate and precise hemodynamic data straight from the source.

The noninvasive approach of the Starling SV provides the information needed to quickly and con dently assess hemodynamic status across the continuum of care

How the Cheetah system works:

4 non-invasive sensor pads are applied to the thorax, creating a 'box' around the heart

A small electric current of known frequency (75kHz) is applied across the thorax between the outer pair of sensors

A voltage signal is recorded between the inner pair of sensors

The flow of blood in the thorax introduces a time delay or phase shift in the signal

Cheetah's proprietary algorithms interpret the signal to provide stroke volume

These signal changes have been correlated to known thermodilution cardiac output in 65,000 patient samples

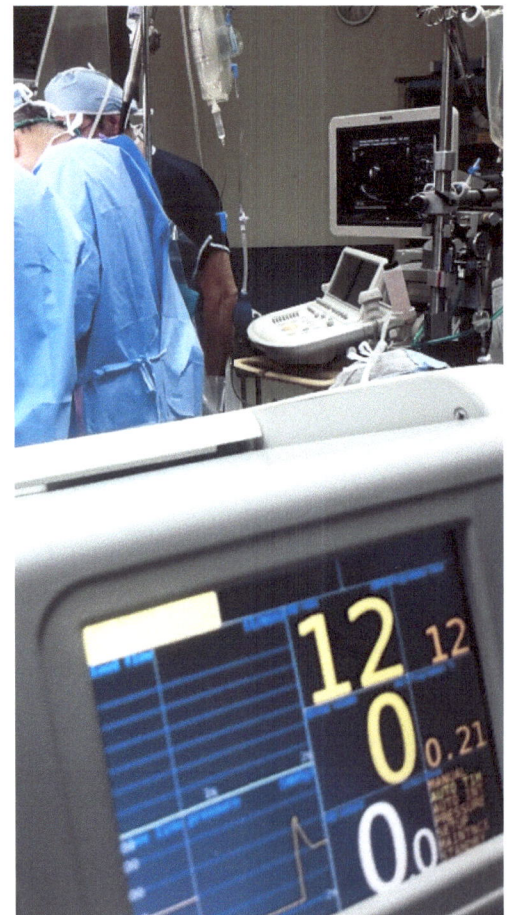

Anesthesia gas machines check list

SETUP	Rationale
1. Verify auxiliary oxygen cylinder and self-inflating manual ventilation device are available & functioning	Failure to be able to ventilate is a major cause of morbidity and mortality related to anesthesia care. Because equipment failure with resulting inability to ventilate the patient can occur at any time, a self-inflating manual ventilation device (eg. AMBU bag) should be present at every anesthetizing location for every case and should be checked for proper function. In addition, a source of oxygen separate from the anesthesia machine and pipeline supply, specifically an oxygen cylinder with regulator and a means to open the cylinder valve, should be immediately available and checked. After checking the cylinder pressure, it is recommended that the main cylinder valve be closed to avoid inadvertent emptying of the cylinder through a leaky or open regulator.
2. Verify patient suction is adequate to clear the airway	Safe anesthetic care requires the immediate availability of suction to clear the airway if needed.

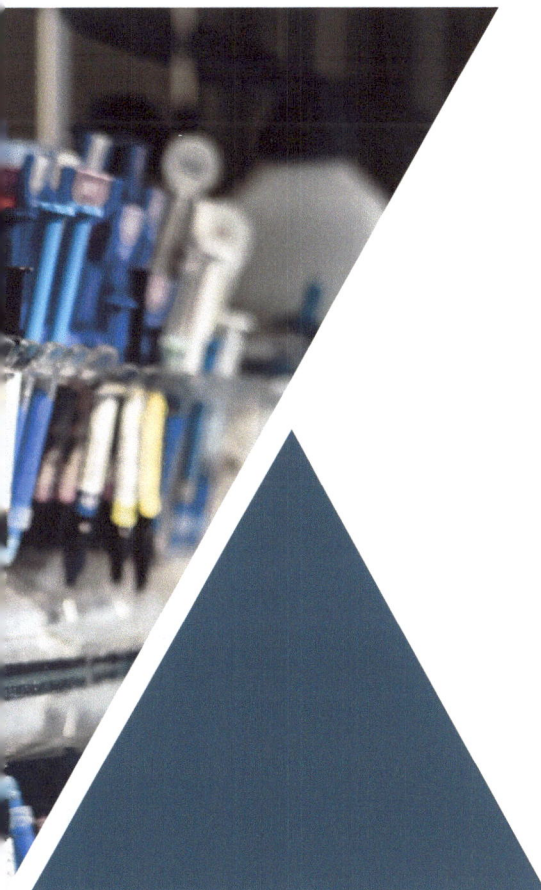

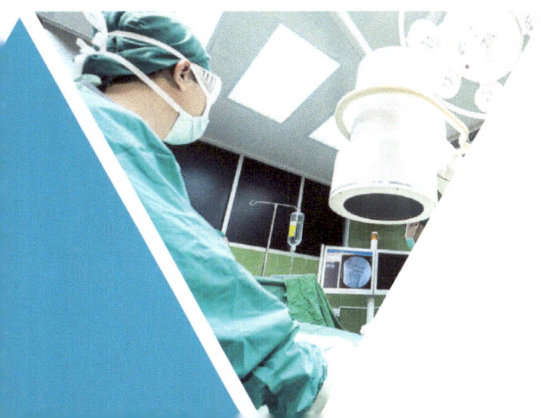

SETUP	Rationale
3. Turn on anesthesia delivery system and confirm that AC power is available.	Anesthesia delivery systems typically function with backup battery power if AC power fails. Unless the presence of AC power is confirmed, the first obvious sign of power failure can be a complete system shutdown when the batteries can no longer power the system. Many anesthesia delivery systems have visual indicators of the power source showing the presence of both AC and battery power. These indicators should be checked and connection of the power cord to a functional AC power source should be confirmed. Desflurane vaporizers require electrical power and recommendations for checking power to these vaporizers should also be followed.
4. Verify availability of required monitors and check alarms.	Standards for patient monitoring during anesthesia are clearly defined. The ability to conform to these standards should be confirmed for every anesthetic. • The first step is to visually verify that the appropriate monitoring supplies (BP cuffs, oximetry probes, etc.) are available. All monitors should be turned on and proper completion of power-up self tests confirmed. • Given the importance of pulse oximetry and capnography to patient safety, verifying proper function of these devices before anesthetizing the patient is essential. ○ Capnometer function can be verified by exhaling through the breathing circuit or gas sensor to generate a capnogram, or verifying that the patient's breathing efforts generate a capnogram before the patient is anesthetized. Visual and audible alarm signals should be generated when this is discontinued.

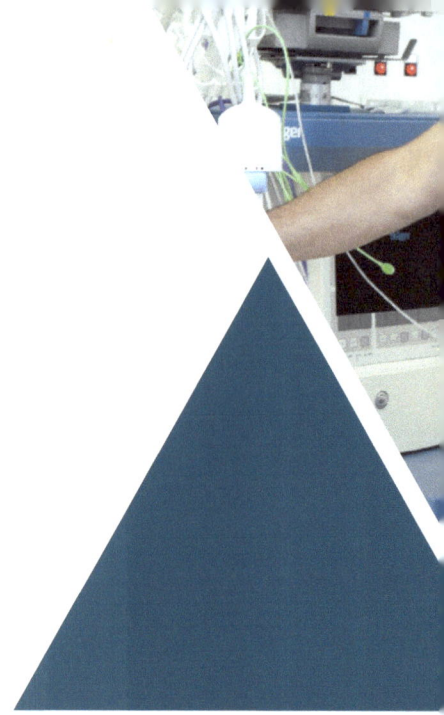

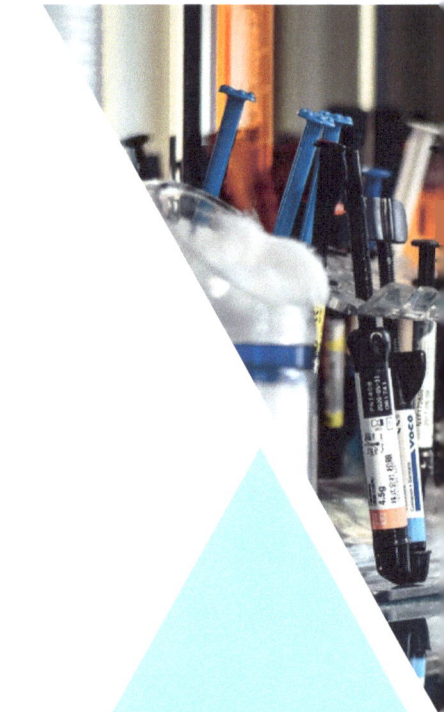

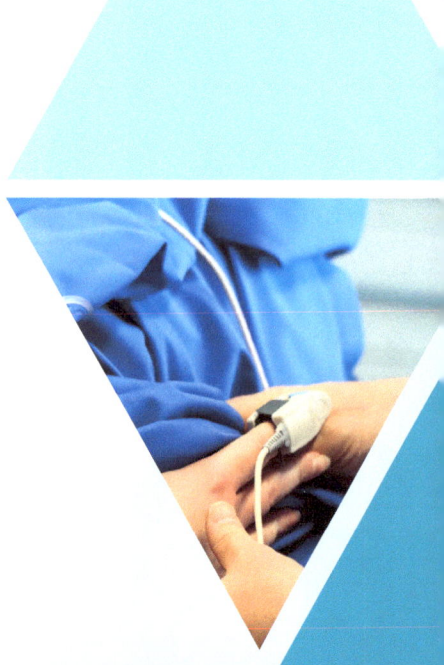

SETUP	Rationale
	○ Pulse oximeter function, including an audible alarm, can be verified by placing the sensor on a finger and observing for a proper recording. The pulse oximeter alarm can be tested by introducing motion artifact or removing the sensor. Audible alarms have also been reconfirmed as essential to patient safety by ASA, AANA, APSF and JCAHO. Proper monitor functioning includes visual and audible alarm signals that function as designed.
5. Verify that pressure is adequate on the spare oxygen cylinder mounted on the anesthesia machine.	Anesthesia delivery systems rely on a supply of oxygen for various machine functions. At a minimum, the oxygen supply is used to provide oxygen to the patient. Pneumatically-powered ventilators also rely on a gas supply. Oxygen cylinder(s) should be mounted on the anesthesia delivery system and determined to have an acceptable minimum pressure. The acceptable pressure depends on the intended use, the design of the anesthesia delivery system and the availability of piped. oxygen. Typically, an oxygen cylinder will be used if the central oxygen supply fails. • If the cylinder is intended to be the primary source of oxygen (e.g. remote site anesthesia), then a cylinder supply sufficient to last for the entire anesthetic is required.

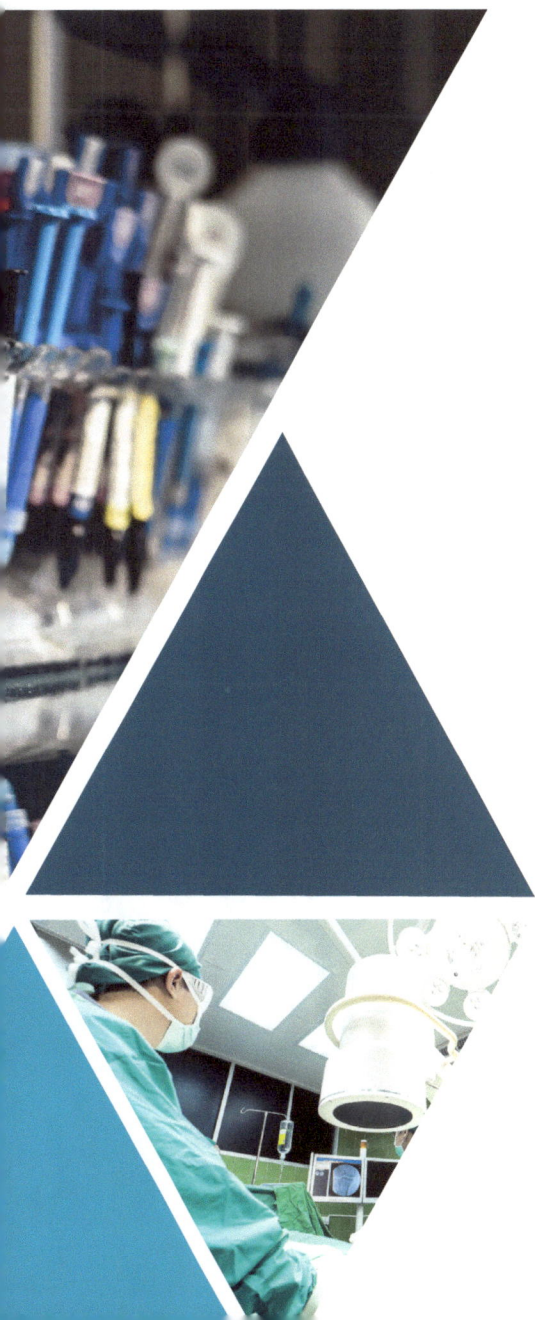

SETUP	Rationale
	• If a pneumatically-powered ventilator that uses oxygen as its driving gas will be used, a full "E" oxygen cylinder may provide only 30 minutes of oxygen. In that case, the maximum duration of oxygen supply can be obtained from an oxygen cylinder if it is used only to provide fresh gas to the patient in conjunction with manual or spontaneous ventilation. Mechanical ventilators will consume the oxygen supply if pneumatically powered ventilators that require oxygen to power the ventilator are used. • Electrically-powered ventilators do not consume oxygen so that the duration of a cylinder supply will depend only on total fresh gas flow. The oxygen cylinder valve should be closed after it has been verified that adequate pressure is present unless the cylinder is to be the primary source of oxygen (i.e. piped oxygen is not available). If the valve remains open and the pipeline supply should fail, the oxygen cylinder can become depleted while the anesthesia provider is unaware of the oxygen supply problem. Other gas supply cylinders (e.g. Heliox, CO2, Air, N2O) need to be checked only if that gas is required to provide anesthetic care.
6. Verify that piped gas pressures are ≥ 50 psig	A minimum gas supply pressure is required for proper function of the anesthesia delivery system. Gas supplied from a central source can fail for a variety of reasons. Therefore the pressure in the piped gas supply should be checked at least once daily.

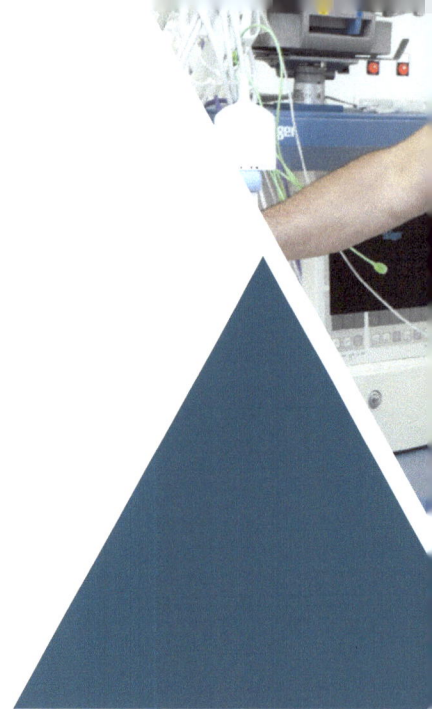

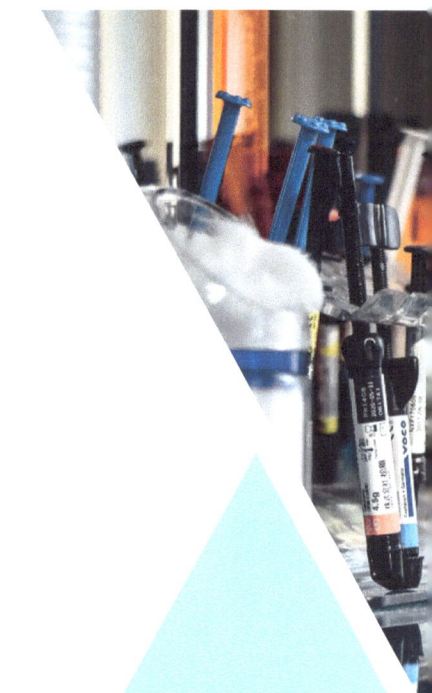

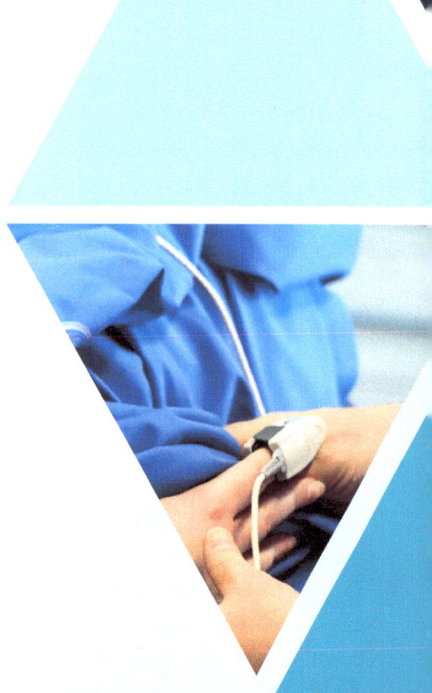

SETUP	Rationale
7. Verify that vaporizers are adequately filled and, if applicable, that the filler ports are tightly closed.	If anesthetic vapor delivery is planned, an adequate supply is essential to reduce the risk of light anesthesia or recall. This is especially true if an anesthetic agent monitor with a low agent alarm is not being used. Partially open filler ports are a common cause of leaks that may not be detected if the vaporizer control dial is not open when a leak test is performed. This leak source can be minimized by tightly closing filler ports. Newer vaporizer designs have filling systems that automatically close the filler port when filling is completed. High and low anesthetic agent alarms are useful to help prevent over- or under-dosage of anesthetic vapor. Use of these alarms is encouraged and they should be set to the appropriate limits and enabled.
8. Verify that there are no leaks in the gas supply lines between the flowmeters and the common gas outlet.	The gas supply in this part of the anesthesia delivery system passes through the anesthetic vaporizer(s) on most anesthesia delivery systems. In order to perform a thorough leak test, each vaporizer must be turned on individually to check for leaks at the vaporizer mount(s) or inside the vaporizer. Furthermore, some machines have a check valve between the flowmeters and the common gas outlet, requiring a negative pressure test to adequately check for leaks.

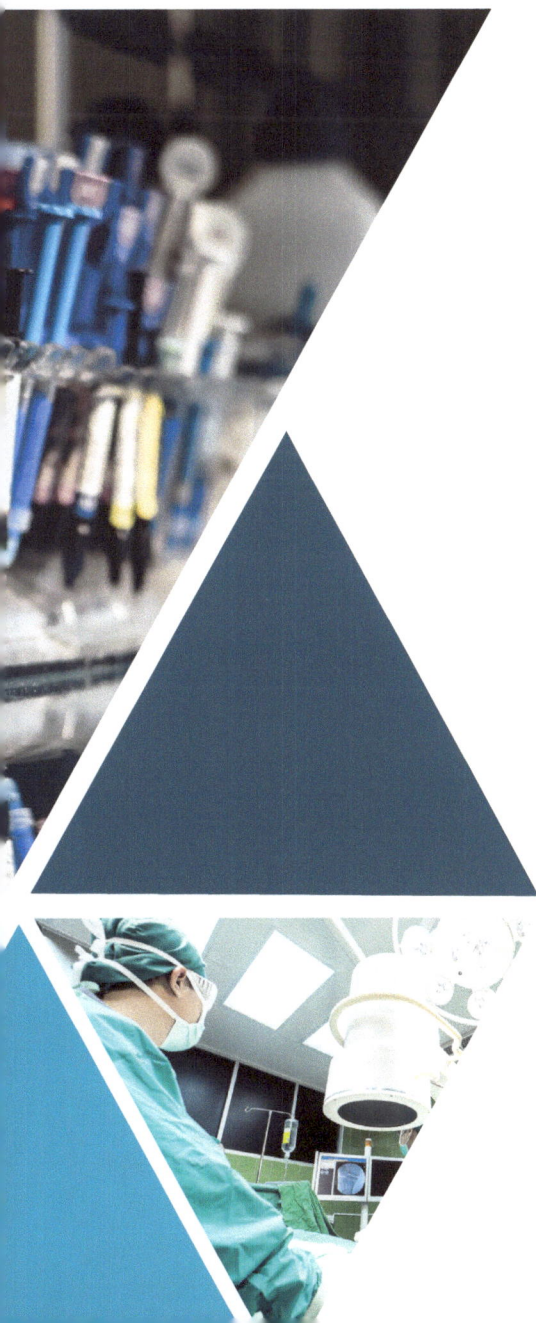

SETUP	Rationale
	Automated checkout procedures typically include a leak test but may not evaluate leaks at the vaporizer especially if the vaporizer is not turned on during the leak test. When relying upon automated testing to evaluate the system for leaks, the automated leak test would need to be repeated for each vaporizer in place. This test should also be completed whenever a vaporizer is changed. The risk of a leak at the vaporizer depends upon the vaporizer design. Vaporizer designs where the filler port closes automatically after filling can reduce the risk of leaks. Technicians can provide useful assistance with this aspect of the machine checkout since it can be time consuming.
9. Test scavenging system function.	A properly functioning scavenging system prevents room contamination by anesthetic gases. • Proper function depends upon correct connections between the scavenging system and the anesthesia delivery system. These connections should be checked daily by a provider or technician. • Depending upon the scavenging system design, proper function may also require that the vacuum level is adequate which should also be confirmed daily. • Some scavenging systems have mechanical positive and negative pressure relief valves. Positive and negative pressure relief is important to protect the patient circuit from pressure fluctuations related to the scavenging system.

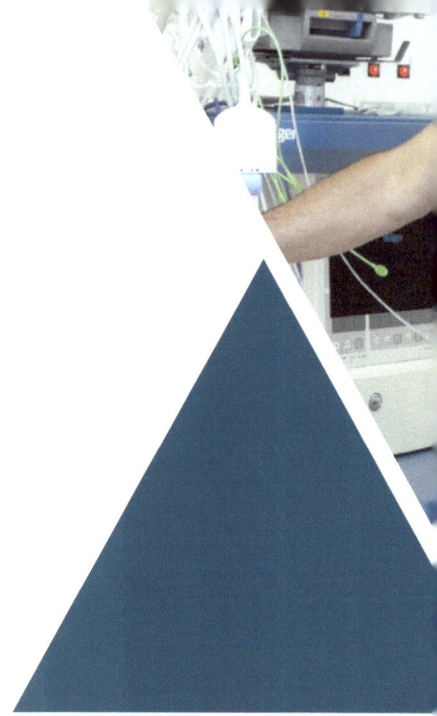

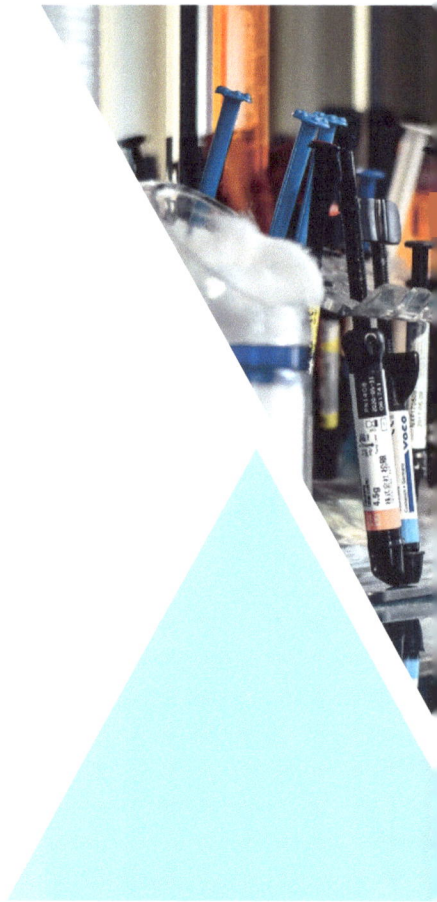

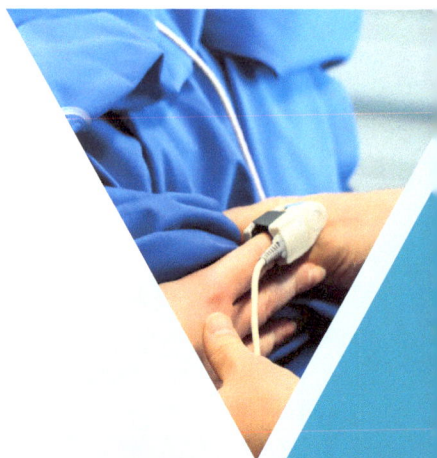

SETUP	Rationale
	Proper checkout of the scavenging system should ensure that positive and negative pressure relief is functioning properly. Due to the complexity of checking for effective positive and negative pressure relief, and the variations in scavenging system design, a properly trained technician can facilitate this aspect of the checkout process.
10. Calibrate, or verify calibration of, the oxygen monitor and check the low oxygen alarm.	Continuous monitoring of the inspired oxygen concentration is the last line of defense against delivering hypoxic gas concentrations to the patient. The oxygen monitor is essential for detecting adulteration of the oxygen supply. • Most oxygen monitors require calibration once daily, although some are self-calibrating. For self-calibrating oxygen monitors, they should be verified to read 21% when sampling room air. This is a step that is easily completed by a trained technician. • When more than one oxygen monitor is present, the primary sensor which will be relied upon for oxygen monitoring should be checked. • The low oxygen concentration alarm should also be checked at this time by setting the alarm above the measured oxygen concentration and confirming that an audible alarm signal is generated.

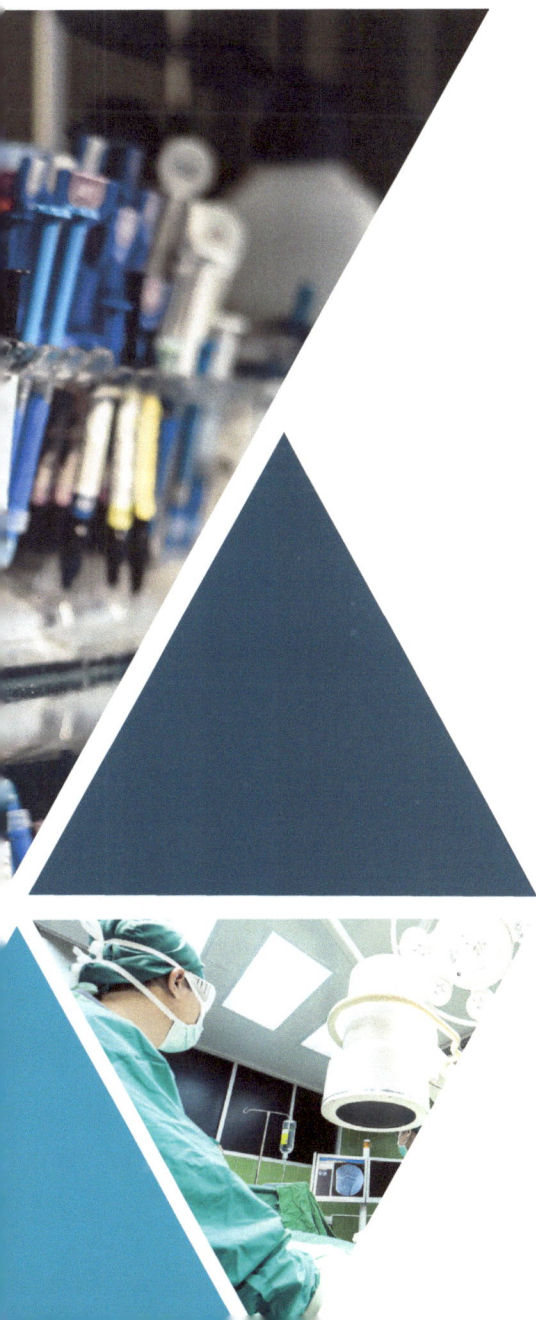

SETUP	Rationale
11. Verify carbon dioxide absorbent is not exhausted.	Proper function of a circle anesthesia system relies on the absorbent to remove carbon dioxide from rebreathed gas. Exhausted absorbent as indicated by the characteristic color change should be replaced. It is possible for absorbent material to lose the ability to absorb CO_2 yet the characteristic color change may be absent or difficult to see. Some newer absorbents do change color when desiccated. Capnography should be utilized for every anesthetic and, when using a circle anesthesia system, rebreathing carbon dioxide as indicated by an inspired CO_2 concentration > 0 can also indicate exhausted absorbent.
12. Breathing system pressure and leak testing.	The breathing system pressure and leak test should be performed with the circuit configuration to be used during anesthetic delivery. If any components of the circuit are changed after this test is completed, the test should be performed again. Although the anesthesia provider should perform this test before each use, anesthesia technicians who replace and assemble circuits can also perform this check and add redundancy to this important checkout procedure. Proper testing will demonstrate that pressure can be developed in the breathing system during both manual and mechanical ventilation and that pressure can be relieved during manual ventilation by opening the APL valve. Automated testing is often implemented in the newer anesthesia delivery systems to evaluate the system for leaks and also to determine the compliance of the breathing system.

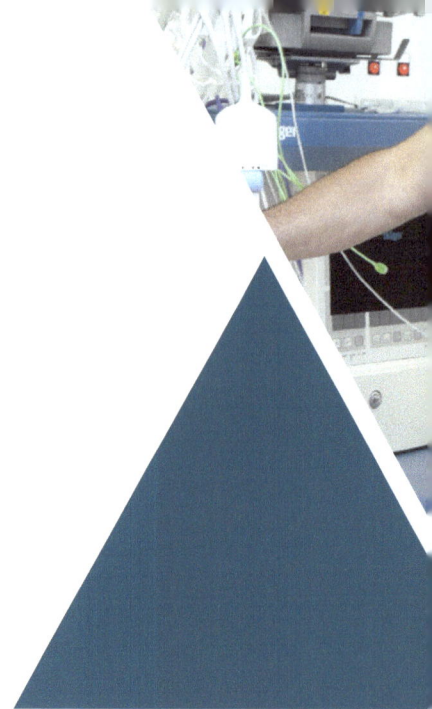

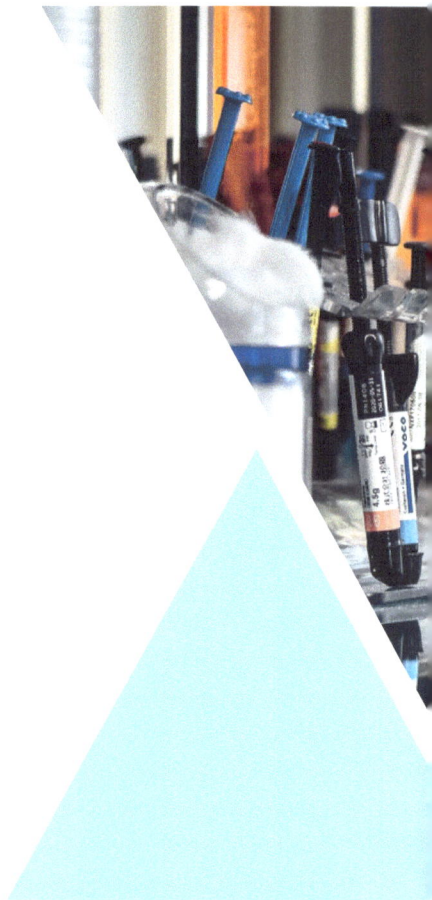

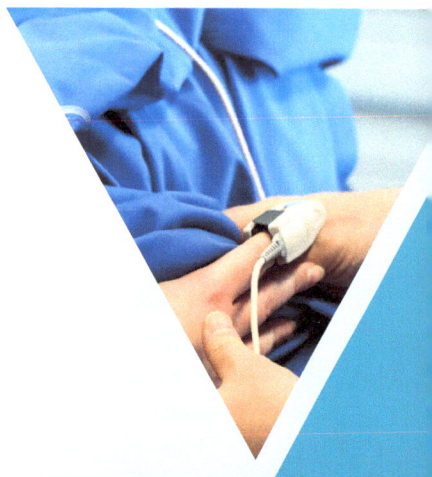

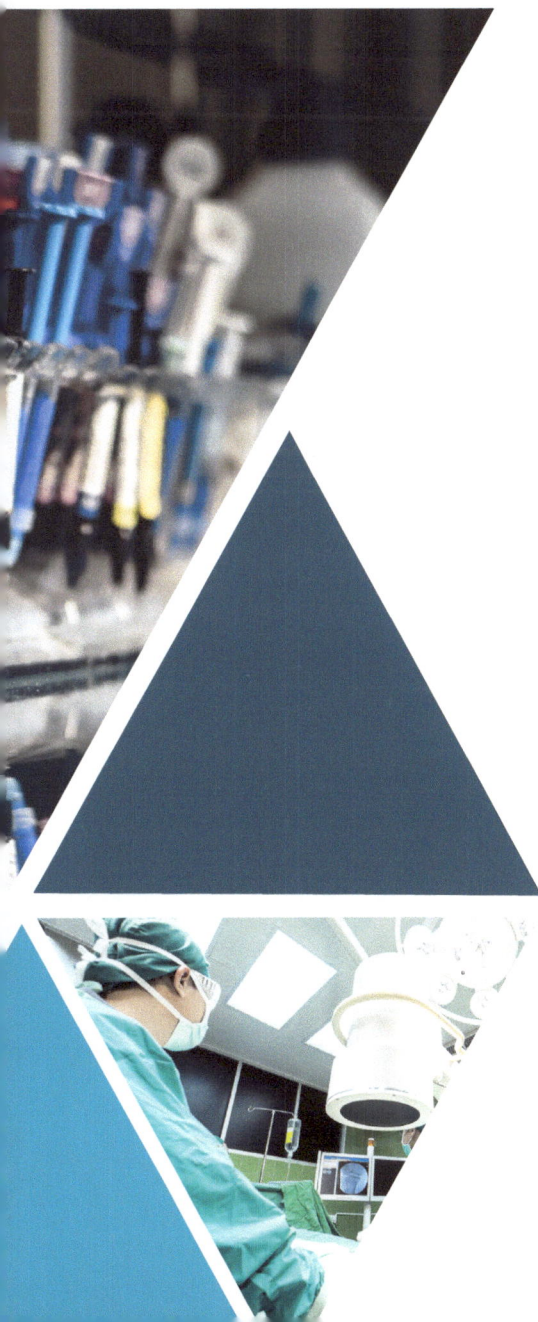

SETUP	Rationale
	The compliance value determined during this testing will be used to automatically adjust the volume delivered by the ventilator to maintain a constant volume delivery to the patient. It is important that the circuit configuration that is to be used be in place during the test.
13. Verify that gas flows properly through the breathing circuit during both inspiration and exhalation.	Pressure and leak testing does not identify all obstructions in the breathing circuit or confirm proper function of the inspiratory and expiratory unidirectional valves. A test lung or second reservoir bag can be used to confirm that flow through the circuit is unimpeded. Complete testing includes both manual and mechanical ventilation. The presence of the unidirectional valves can be assessed visually during the PAC. Proper function of these valves cannot be visually assessed since subtle valve incompetence may not be detected. Checkout procedures to identify valve incompetence which may not be visually obvious can be implemented but are typically too complex for daily testing. A trained technician can perform regular valve competence tests. Capnography should be used during every anesthetic and the presence of carbon dioxide in the inspired gases can help to detect an incompetent valve.

SETUP	Rationale
14. Document completion of checkout procedures	Each individual responsible for checkout procedures should document completion of these procedures. Documentation gives credit for completing the job and can be helpful if an adverse event should occur. Some automated checkout systems maintain an audit trail of completed checkout procedures that are dated and timed.
15. Confirm ventilator settings and evaluate readiness to deliver anesthesia care. (ANESTHESIA TIME OUT)	This step is intended to avoid errors due to production pressure or other sources of haste. The goal is to confirm that appropriate checks have been completed and that essential equipment is indeed available. The concept is analogous to the "time out" used to confirm patient identity and surgical site prior to incision. Improper ventilator settings can be harmful especially if a small patient is following a much larger patient or vice versa. Pressure limit settings (when available) should be used to prevent excessive volume delivery from improper ventilator settings. Items to check: • Monitors functional? • Capnogram present? • Oxygen saturation by pulse oximetry measured? • Flowmeter and ventilator settings proper? • Manual/ventilator switch set to manual? • Vaporizer(s) adequately filled?

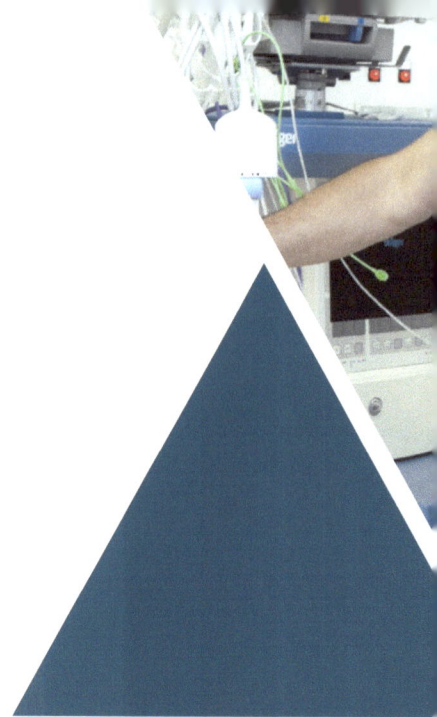

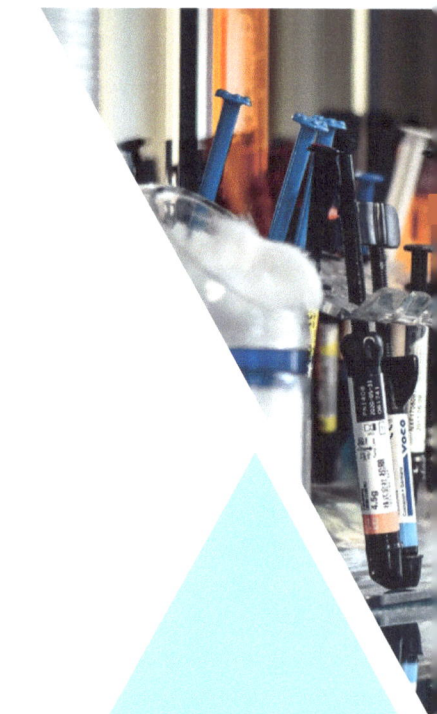

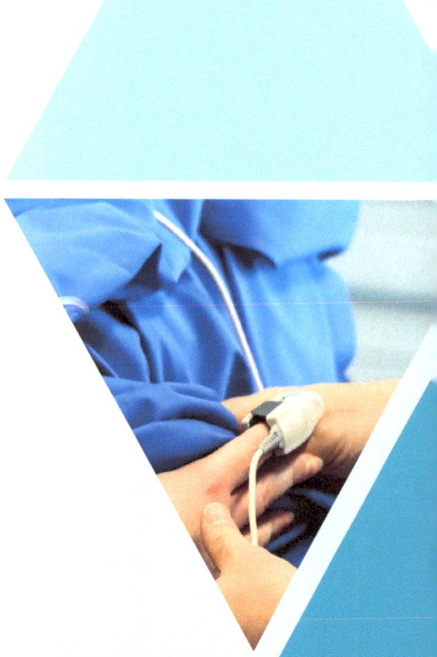

SETUP	Rationale
Timing	Perform the entire checklist daily. Repeat the following items before each case: • 2: Verify patient suction is adequate to clear the airway • 4: Verify availability of required monitors, including alarms. • 7: Verify that vaporizers are adequately filled and if applicable that the filler ports are tightly closed. • 11: Verify carbon dioxide absorbent is not exhausted • 12: Breathing system pressure and leak testing. • 13: Verify that gas flows properly through the breathing circuit during both inspiration and exhalation. • 14: Document completion of checkout procedures. • 15: Confirm ventilator settings and evaluate readiness to deliver anesthesia care. (ANESTHESIA TIME OUT)

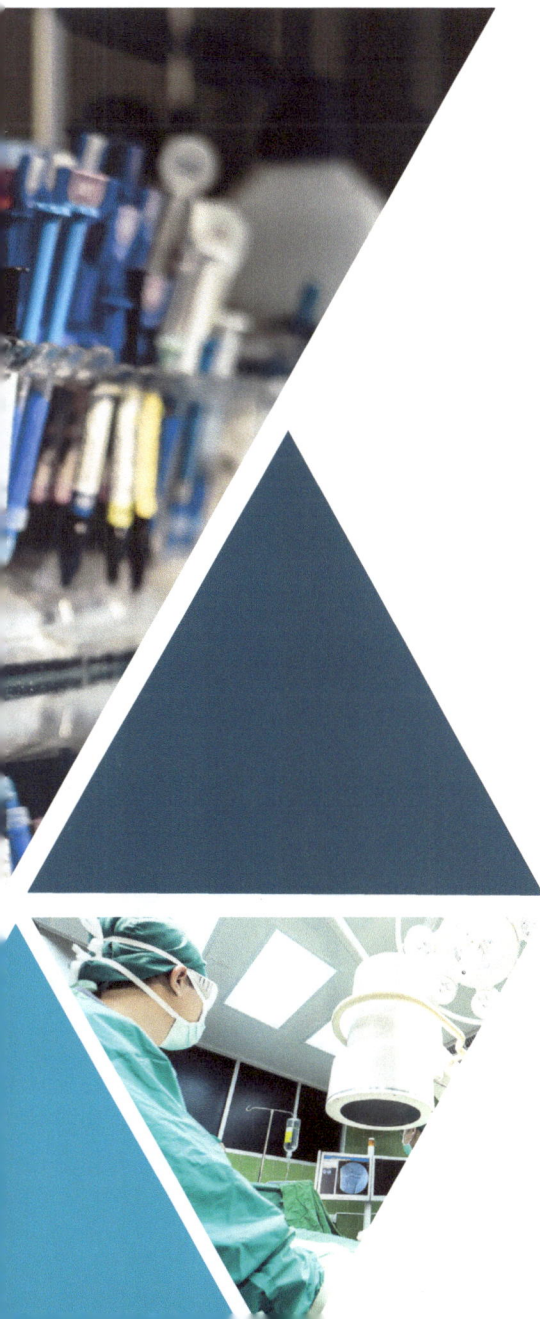

HIGH PRESSURE LEAK TEST

Leaks can come from a few places, and the main ones are the canister and the hoses. For this reason, the machine should be checked daily for leaks. If any leaks are discovered, they should be addressed immediately. There is a basic leak test you can do. Start by closing the pop-off valve, then put your thumb over the end of the anesthesia hose. Press the oxygen flush valve to fill the reservoir bag to a pressure of 20 centimeters.

Then, just wait a few seconds to see if the needle on the pressure gauge drops. If it does, then you have a leak. You can check two bags at once by using a second one instead of your thumb. Place a bag at the end of the hose instead of blocking it with your thumb. Push the oxygen flush valve to fill both bags to 20 centimeters. After checking your anesthesia machine for leaks, any problems should be addressed right away. This should be done before every shift in the interest of patient safety and the performance of the machine.

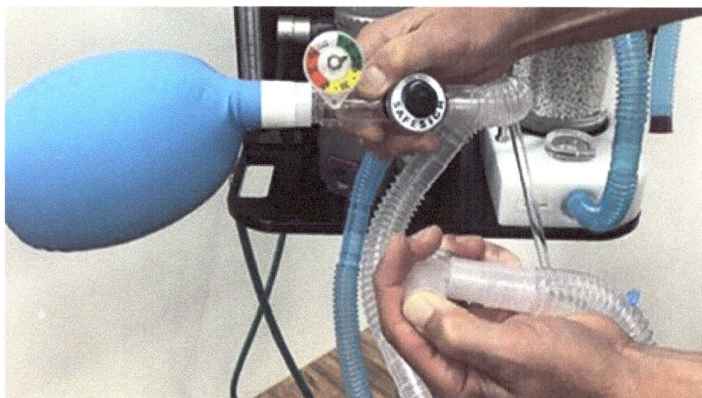

Electronic checklists

Regardless of the model of gas machine, users must be able to answer at least three patient safety questions affirmatively upon completion of the electronic or automatic portion of the checklist:

1. **(Oxygen check)** Is there oxygen in the oxygen line?
   - Ensure that inspired oxygen reads 21%, with sample line open to air
   - Ensure that this reading goes up when the breathing circuit is reassembled, and the flush is pushed for a high-pressure leak test.
2. **(Leak Check)** Is the reassembled circuit free of leaks? Can I give a breath?
   - Remember to do high-pressure check after everything reassembled and checkout finished (If gas analysis tubing falls off, there will be a leak)
3. **(Flow Check)** Can they take a breath, and exhale it?
   - Use a second bag attached at the elbow as a test lung, or breathe through the circuit.
   - Ensure that gas flows in a tidal (to-and-fro) manner between bellows and test lung, and between manual breathing bag and test lung.
   - Visually observe that the unidirectional valves in the breathing circuit are working.
   - Confirm that there is no obstruction to inhalation or exhalation (no mold flash or plastic emboli obstructing the circuit).

_____

The newer machines (Apollo, Perseus, Fabius, Aisys) have system checkout routines that are electronic and automated. The operator follows instructions to activate flows of gases, occlude the breathing circuit during the leak check, switch from manual to mechanical ventilation, open and close the pop off valve, and manually check various functions (suction, or emergency oxygen cylinder supply). All these machine checklists require users to check certain aspects on their own, and these aspects vary from machine to machine, which creates a need for training on each machine anesthetists use.

Local departments must create checklist procedures for each type of gas machine they own. Electronic checklists can be expected to cover most or all the steps of the PAC 2008, but this is apparent only after some study, because each checklist differs in important respects. Models may differ on whether (or how) they check oxygen monitoring, vaporizer leaks, etc. You can see samples posted at Sample PAC procedures. Electronic checklists may (e.g. Aisys) require that the gas analysis aspiration sampling line is disconnected before the breathing circuit is occluded by attaching it to a post. Apollo requires that the sampling line remains connected. Electronic checklists may (or may not) require the operator to repeat leak tests with each vaporizer turned on.

Electronic system checkout is logged, but may be bypassed in an emergency. Though the normal morning checklist takes only 5-8 minutes, the operator can perform other tasks simultaneously (such as filling syringes), so it does not appreciably slow morning preparation, unless one had not been accustomed to performing a morning gas machine checklist at all.

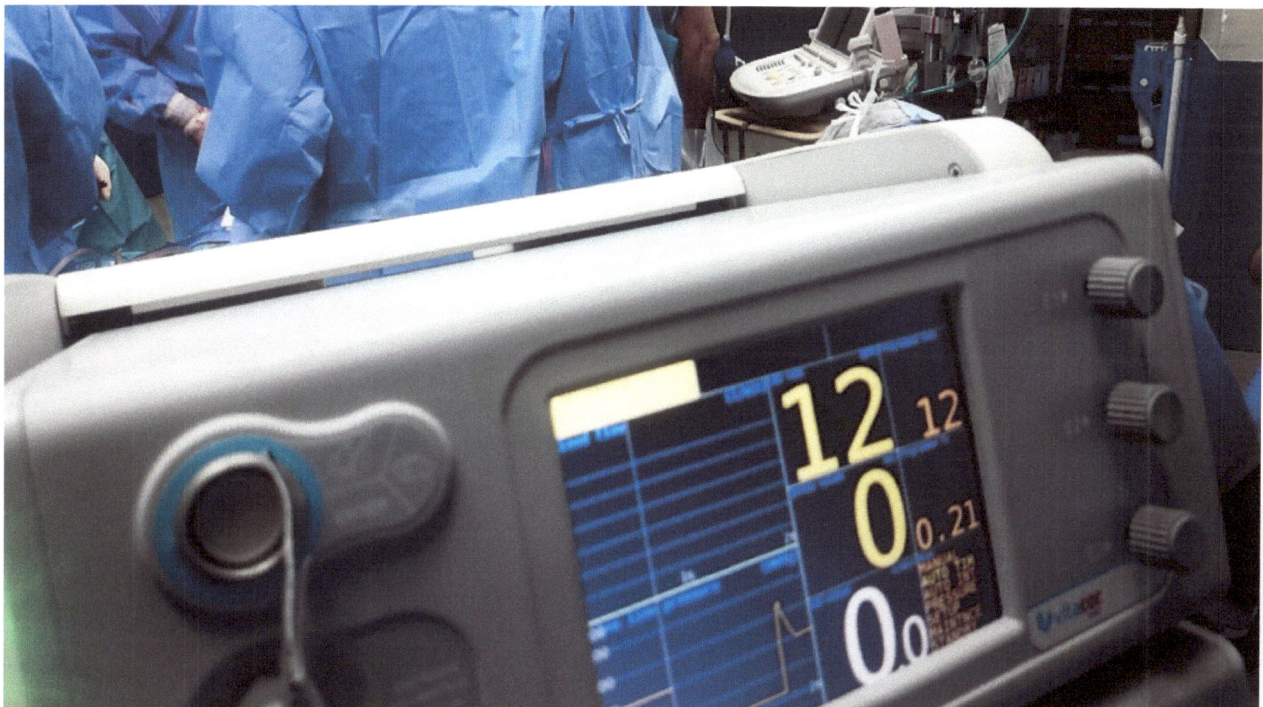

AWS (Anesthesia Workstation) Quick-Check & PaF test

As anesthesia techs it is not enough to understand the anesthesia gas machine we must also understand our anesthesia providers and what their general needs and wants as well as specific case needs are. Recently a quick protocol to ensure readiness was proposed (Anesth Analg 2019;129:1439). The AWS-QUICKcheck verifies 4 things. It is performed as each patient is brought to the OR, during pre-oxygenation, and just after induction agents:

1. **Is a bag-valve-mask available?** If ventilation difficulty, it can distinguish whether problems are in patient, or breathing circuit.
2. **Is suction available?**
3. **Is the anesthetic circuit functioning correctly, by and large?** Proven by the "Pressure and Flow-Test" (PaF test) before connecting the patient, and by observing/palpating the breathing bag during preoxygenation, which ensures:
   - Adequate flow of oxygen
   - Good mask fit (very important)
   - The patient is breathing
   - The circuit is unobstructed
   - The Bag/Vent switch is on "Bag" not "Vent" (older machines)
4. **Is the desired FIO2 being delivered?**
5. **Are the lungs ventilated?** (check end tidal CO2, and also the feel of the bag during manual ventilation just after intubation of the trachea.

PaF test

Pressure and Flow (PaF) check combines leak check (step 12) and flow check (step 13). It is performed before the patient is connected and takes only a few seconds.

- **"Pressure" test**
  - Set APL valve to approximately 30 mbar, occlude the elbow, fill the reservoir bag with oxygen flush, and squeeze the bag. No visible, tactile, or audible leak should be observed.
- **"Flow" test**
  - Then the patient opening is released, and gas has to exhaust audibly (onomatopoeic "paff") indicating forward flow.
  - Replace your thumb, repressurize the bag, and open the APL. Pressure should be released into the scavenger indicating backward flow

While there is no universally accepted machine checklist less than the full PAC, situations do arise in anesthesia (e.g. for trauma or emergency cesarean section) where there is neither time nor opportunity to fully check the anesthesia gas machine. The PAC 2008 states "The PAC is essential to safe care, but should not delay initiating care if the patient needs are so urgent that time taken to complete the PAC could worsen the patient's outcome."

Building in good habits as you start every anesthetic will help you during emergencies. This includes:

- Check for Ambu and suction as you enter the room and apply monitors.

- PaF (leak & flow) test before placing the mask on any patients face, every time.

- Observing during pre-oxygenation: bag movement, oxygen flowmeter, FIO2, capnograph.

With all new machines, the electronic checklist can be bypassed in emergencies. Whether the quick minimum test above is acceptable must be determined by each clinical practice. It has been suggested that workstations be left on if trauma or obstetric cases must be done on a moment's notice (Anesthesiology 2001;95:567). The Aisys checklist can be bypassed an indefinite number of times, but it will display a visible message until the electronic checkout is performed.

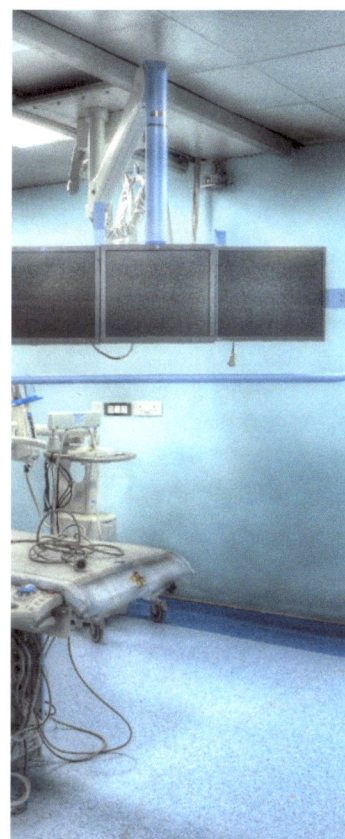

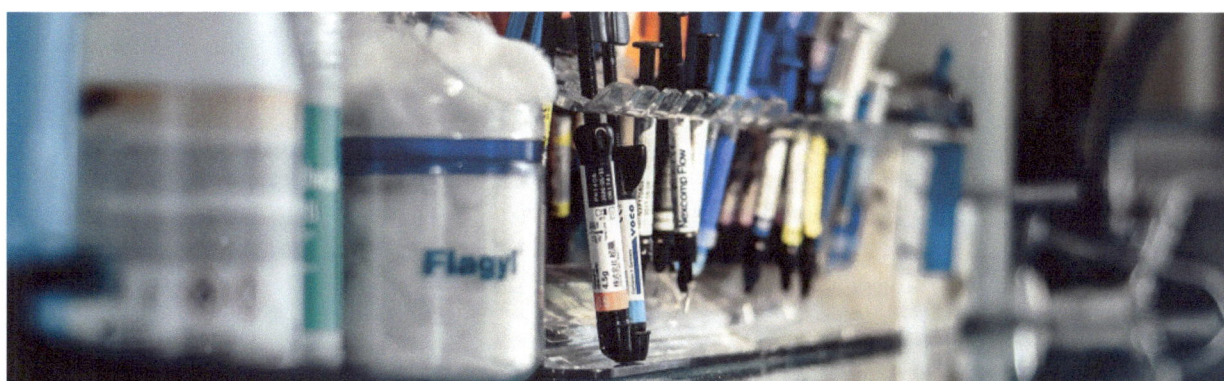

CHECKLIST FOR OLDER ANESTHESIA GAS MACHINES

Introduction The anesthesia gas machine must be equipped with an ascending bellows ventilator and certain monitors (capnograph, pulse oximeter, oxygen analyzer, spirometer, breathing system pressure monitor with high and low pressure alarms). If not so equipped, the checklist must be modified.

1. *Verify backup ventilation equipment is available & functioning.*

- Contaminated oxygen supply, loss of oxygen supply pressure, and obstruction of the breathing system, though rare, cause the machine to be totally inoperable. So check for that Ambu!

2. *Check oxygen cylinder supply*

   a. One cylinder must be at least half full (1000 psi).

   b. It is not necessary to:

      - Check any other cylinders beside oxygen

      - "Bleed" the pressure off the cylinder pressure gauge after checking

   c. Leave cylinder closed after checking.

   d. While you're behind the machine, check suction, Ambu bag and extra circuit present. Also: gas analysis scavenged, scavenger caps all present, location of circuit breakers, any loose pipeline, electrical, or etc. connections, head strap, tank wrench, and color/date of CO_2 absorbent.

3. *Check central pipeline supplies.*

   o Check for proper connection at wall

   o Check the pipeline pressure gauge- should read approximately 50 psi.

   o It is not necessary to unhook pipeline connections at wall.

4. *Check initial status of low pressure system.*

   o Remove oxygen analyzer sensor and begin calibration.

   o Check liquid level and fill vaporizers if necessary; fill ports tightly capped.

   o Check vaporizer interlock.

CHECKLIST FOR OLDER ANESTHESIA GAS MACHINES

5. *Perform leak check of low pressure system.*

- Leaks as low as 100 mL/min may lead to critical decrease in the concentration of volatile anesthetic (creating a risk for intraoperative awareness), or permit hypoxic mixtures under certain circumstances.
- Negative pressure leak test (10 sec.) is recommended.
- Repeat for each vaporizer.

6. *Turn master switch on.*

7. *Test flowmeters.*

- Check for damage, full range, hypoxic guard.

8. *Calibrate oxygen monitor*

- Final line of defense against hypoxic mixtures. Trust it until you can prove it wrong. Mandatory for all general anesthetics, or whenever using the breathing circuit (for example during sedation)
- Calibrate/daily check: expose to room air and allow to equilibrate (2 min). Then expose to oxygen source and ensure it reads near 100%

9. *Check initial status of breathing system*

- Assemble circuit with all accessories.

10. *Test ventilation systems and unidirectional valves (Flow Check)*

- Test ventilator, observe action of unidirectional valves, ensure gas flows properly in circuit without obstruction.

11. *Perform leak check of breathing system*

- The "usual" high pressure check.
- Let the gas out of the circuit through the Popoff (APL) valve, not the elbow.

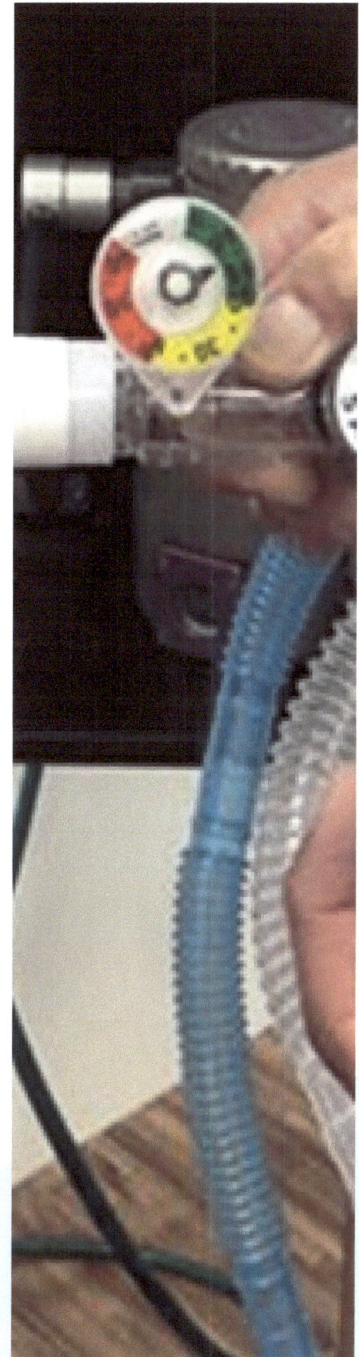

Negative pressure leak check for older machines

nidirectional valves (check valves) are present in some machines between the vaporizers and the common gas outlet. Without them (or internal vaporizer design modifications), the cycling of positive pressure in the breathing circuit leads to increases in vaporizer output (the pumping effect). A high pressure check of the breathing circuit will not detect leaks upstream of these valves, since the high pressure in the breathing circuit will only be transmitted upstream to the check valve, and no further. These upstream areas are vulnerable areas. Glass flowtubes, internal vaporizer seals, and rubber O-rings are susceptible to failure.

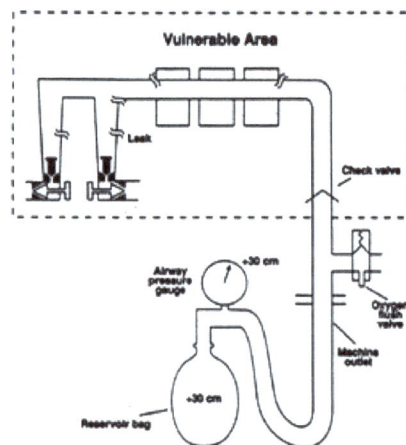

Negative pressure leak check

negative pressure leak check that will work on any older anesthesia machine. Unfortunately, this step is somewhat archaic; thus, not well-understood or practiced often enough, in part due to its reliance on an accessory suction bulb, which is meant to be applied to the common gas outlet. The bulb is pumped until it flattens: it will remain flat if no internal leaks are present proximal to the common gas outlet. The test is repeated with each vaporizer turned on.

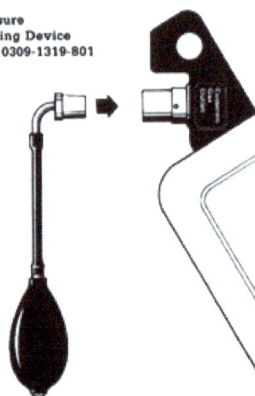

This test cannot be done on modern machines (where the common gas outlet is inaccessible). Apollo uses negative pressure as part of its electronic self-test; Aisys and Fabius do not.

Cleaning and sterilization

It is controversial whether equipment like breathing circuits can transmit infection. Most, if not all, would agree that sterilization is essential after use on a patient with known or suspected infection of the respiratory tract, especially with virulent organisms. Likewise, we should protect compromised patients from contamination arising from our equipment. In any case, handwashing between patients, as well as universal precautions, are mandatory in anesthetic practice.

Cleaning equipment means removal of foreign matter without special attempts to kill microorganisms. Equipment should be pre-rinsed as soon as possible after use to prevent drying of organic material; then soaked, removal of soil, rinsing and drying.

Sterilization

Moist heat methods

- Pasteurization (less than 100 degrees C) disinfects but doesn't sterilize (destroys many but not all organisms).
- Boiling kills all forms of bacteria, most spores, practically all viruses if boiled at least 30 minutes.
- Autoclaving (steam sterilization under pressure) kills all bacteria, spores and viruses.

Liquid sterilization

Useful for heat sensitive equipment, but recontamination possible during drying and re-wrapping. Of several agents (chlorhexidine [Hibitane®], phenolic compounds, hexachlorophene, ethyl or isopropyl alcohols), glutaraldehyde is the only one effective against both tubercule bacillus and viruses, but its vapors are a health hazard.

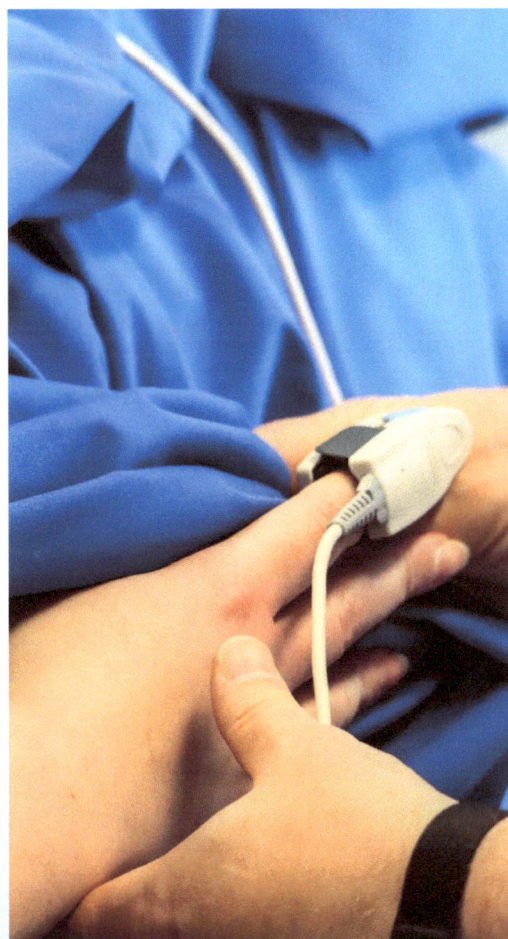

Chemical gas sterilization

Ethylene oxide (ETO) is a synthetic gas widely used, especially for heat or moisture-sensitive items like rubber and plastic. Kills bacteria, spores, fungi, larger viruses. Can be various patient reactions if not aerated (in wrapper) sufficiently after ETO exposure. The gas is also explosive and toxic.

Other means

Gamma radiation kills all bacteria, spores and viruses. Used for sterilization of disposable equipment - not practical for everyday needs of hospitals.

Care of specific equipment

- **Carts & gas machine** - wipe top, front, sides with detergent/germicide (D/G) daily and place a clean covering on top; clean entire cart inside and out weekly or after contaminated cases
- **Breathing circuits, ETT, face masks, airways, resuscitation bags-** generally single use, or follow department policy & manufacturer's guidelines
- **Absorber, unidirectional valves, relief valve, bellows -** follow manufacturer's instructions, use autoclavable components or filters on the circle system for known infected cases
- **Blades, Magills-** cleanse, sterilization, store clean
- **Headstraps, BP cuffs -** Items in contact with intact skin need periodic cleansing, or should be cleansed if soiled

The Centers for Disease Control has a collection of useful information relating to bloodborne diseases and universal precautions.

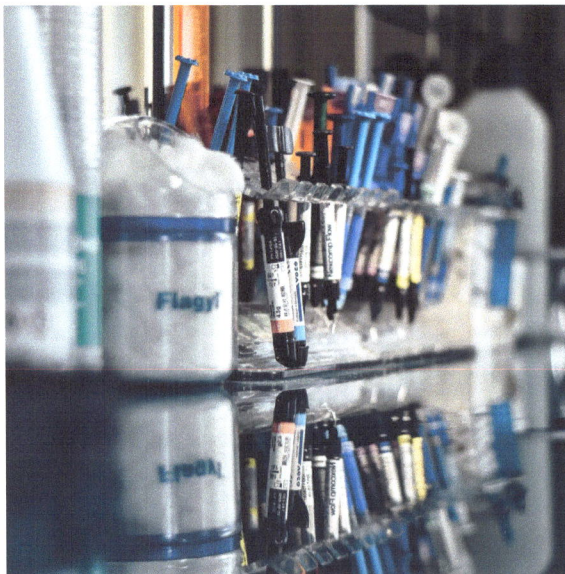

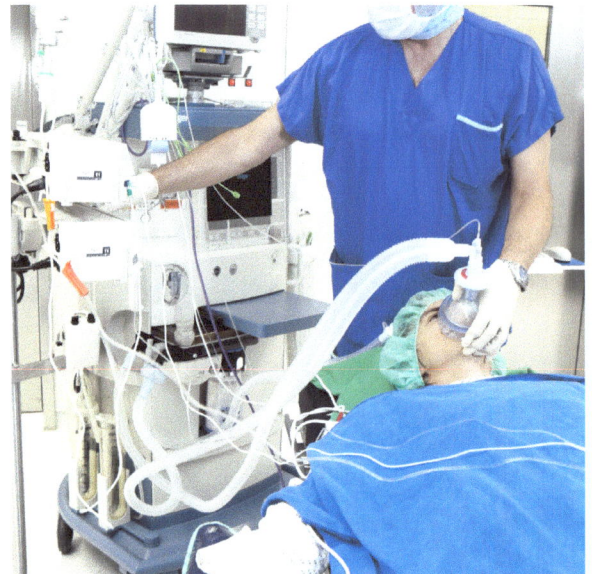

Using the anesthesia workstation as a ventilator for critically ill patients-Technical considerations

Michael Dosch CRNA PhD Revised March 31, 2020

Who should run the anesthesia workstation

Should anesthesia workstations be used as ventilators for the critically ill?

- All manufacturers caution that the use is off-label, and the responsibility lies with the user. All offer guidance because the current situation is unprecedented.[1–3] The US Food & Drug Administration has given authorization for emergency use.[4,5] The ASA (American Society of Anesthesiologists) & APSF (Anesthesia Patient Safety Foundation) have authored joint guidance for use in critically ill patients.[6]

Anesthesia providers should set up, check, and manage the anesthesia workstation.

- GE- "There is a risk of serious injury or death if the devices are not used by properly trained clinicians, continuously monitored, and used in accordance with the instructions for use... The devices are intended to be used by clinicians who are trained in the administration of general anesthesia. There are unique characteristics that differentiate anesthesia devices from standard ICU ventilators... All users should be familiar with the anesthesia system user interface, controls, functions, configurations, alarms, and theory of operation before using these devices."[1] "Because anesthesia devices are designed as attended devices, most anesthesia devices do not continue ventilation... in the event of a critical device malfunction."[1]

- Drager & Mindray offer similar guidance.[2,3] ASA/APSF state "An anesthesia professional should be immediately available at all times (24/7/365) to manage the use of the anesthesia machine as an ICU ventilator. Intensivists, ICU nurses, and respiratory therapists are not trained to manage anesthesia machines and are likely to be overextended and stressed. Consultation with intensivists on the preferred ventilation strategy is of course desirable."[6]

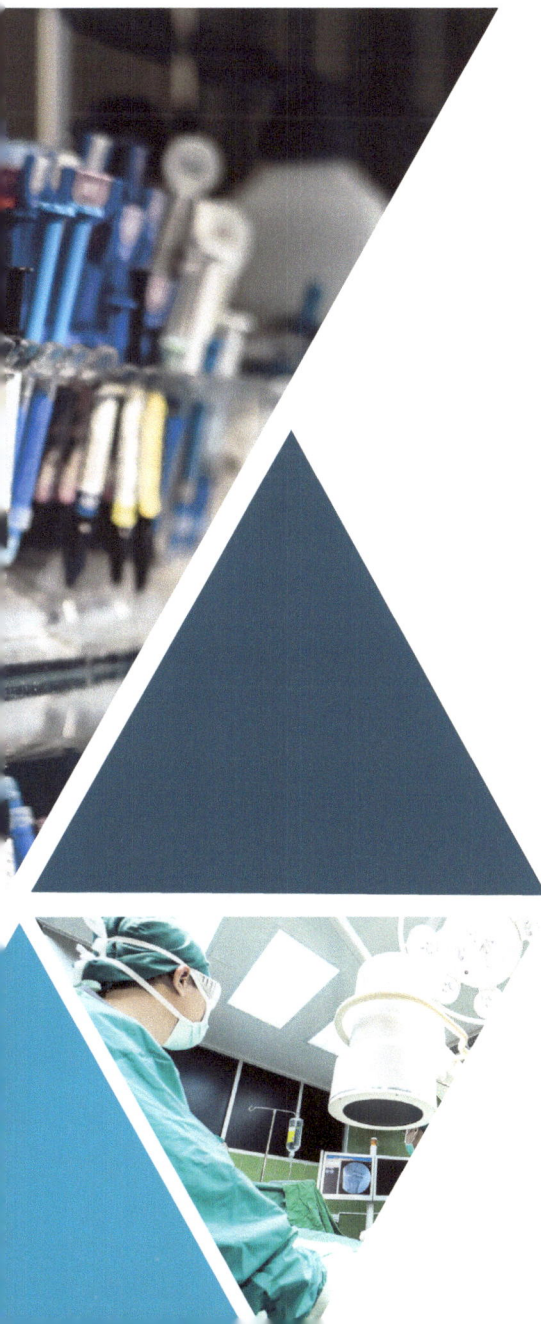

Anesthesia providers must be in constant attendance or immediately available to respond to alarms and make appropriate adjustments.

- GE "Anesthesia devices are designed and intended to be fully attended/monitored devices, which requires a clinician to be in proximity of the device at all times. This is different from the potential use case in ICU ventilation. It is critical to ensure the proper use and continuous monitoring of the anesthesia device function and ventilation is maintained... Anesthesia systems are designed for use in an attended environment. Device audio alert levels (volume) may not be adequate for the ICU use environment. Ensure the device audio level is adequate for the ICU or provide alternative methods of continual status monitoring. The anesthesia machines do not have the ability to generate alerts via the hospital nurse call alarm systems."[1]

- Drager & Mindray offer similar guidance.[2,3] "The user interface of Dräger anesthesia devices cannot be protected against non-authorized users. Therefore, the operating organization must ensure that non-authorized users cannot approach the device to avoid the settings being changed, or therapy is stopped (no alarm is generated when the device is switched to standby)... The alarm and safety concept of Dräger anesthesia is designed for a permanent presence of the user within a distance of up to four meters... remote supervision (e.g. via central station) is not sufficient."[2]

- ASA/APSF "Anesthesia professionals will be needed to put these machines into service and to manage them while in use. Safe and effective use requires an understanding of the capabilities of the machines available, the differences between anesthesia machines and ICU ventilators, and how to set anesthesia machine controls to mimic ICU-type ventilation strategies."[6]

Breathing circuit

Fresh gas flow (FGF)-

- The lower fresh gas flows that anesthesia providers are accustomed to (1-2 L/min) are advantageous in short-term ventilation, by conserving tracheal heat and humidity, and giving economy of volatile agents. For chronic ventilation, lower FGF may cause excessive water vapor in the circuit, and condensation. This may interfere with flow sensors, the accuracy of tidal volume delivery, and trigger additional breaths (as exhalations bubble through collected water in the expiratory limb).

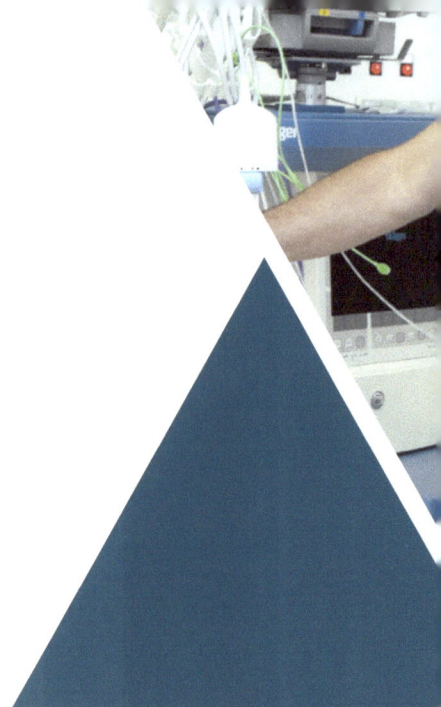

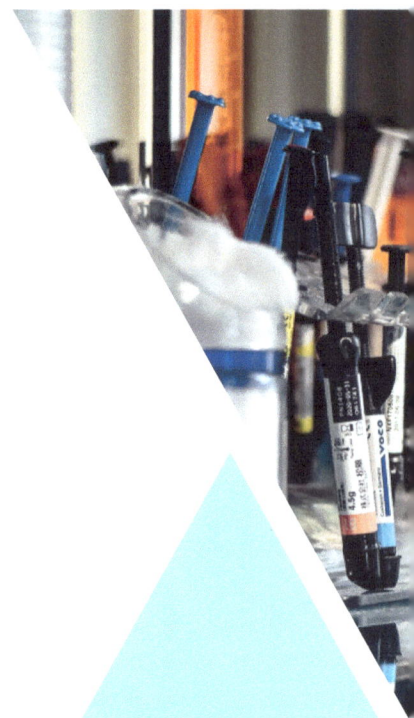

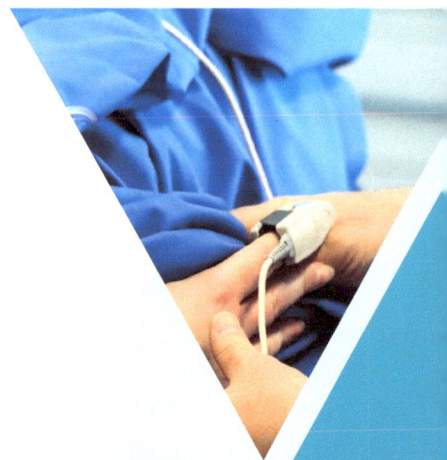

Higher FGF uses a large amount of oxygen and dries the tracheal mucosa. For these reasons, manufacturers have suggested fresh gas flows of:

- GE- 50% or more of patient's minute ventilation (VE = VT x RR)[1]

- Drager- 150% of VE[2]
- Mindray- 100% of VE[3]

- If using lower FGF, **increase FGF > VE for15 min every four hours** to help dry the internal components of the circuit[6]

N2O & Vaporizers-

The use of nitrous oxide or vaporized anesthetics is not recommended.[1-3,6] It is advised that vaporizers be removed to prevent triggering malignant hyperthermia, among other reasons. "Anesthesia machines have the capability of providing inhaled anesthetics for sedation during long-term care. While this might be an attractive option if intravenous sedatives are in short supply, it is not generally recommended when the machines are used as ICU ventilators. Certainly, this is not advised without proper waste anesthetic gas scavenging which will typically only be available in the OR. The potentially detrimental effects of long-term sedation with inhaled anesthetics have not been studied. Provision of inhaled anesthesia would require the constant presence of an anesthesia provider at the bedside to monitor the physiologic effects." [6]

Scavenging

In addition to the above, it is recommended that" Scavenging is not required or necessary if appropriate viral filters are placed on the circuits... Suction outlets are available in the ICU but cannot be attached to the WAGD [Waste Anesthesia Gas Disposal] connection on the machine due to connector incompatibility."[6]

Suctioning

Switch to Manual/Spontaneous ("bag" mode) during tracheal suctioning.[1]

Conserving humidity, oxygen, carbon dioxide absorbent-

Humidity is conserved by the use of lower FGF, and by using a heat moisture exchange filter (HMEF) at the Y junction of the breathing circuit.6 Active humidification is not recommended. Users should be vigilant for accumulation of water in circuit hoses and monitor water traps, HMEFs, and condensers if present.

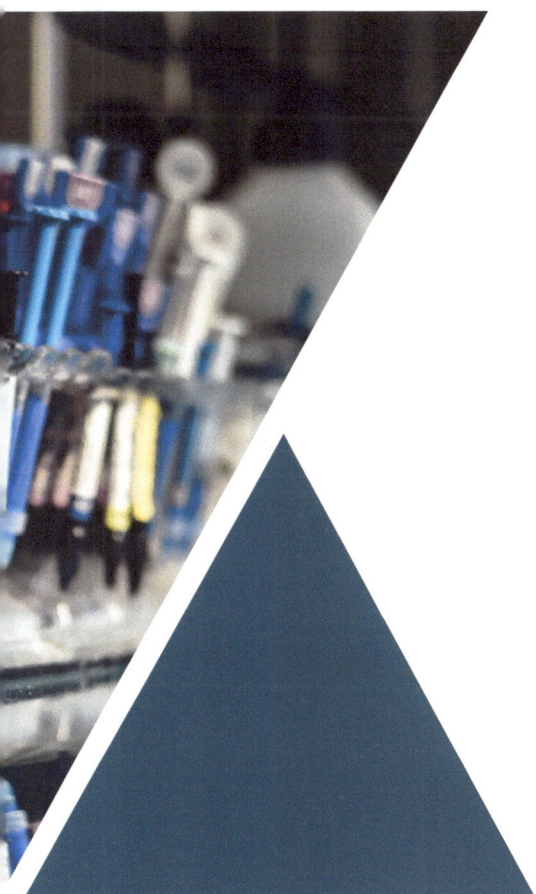

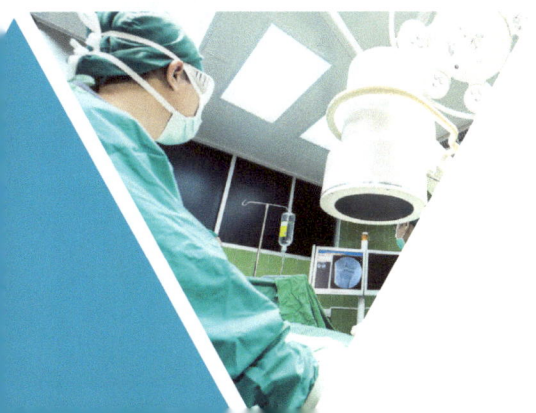

- Oxygen may be conserved by low FGF, by using a workstation with an electrically-powered bellows (Drager) rather than a gas-powered bellows (GE), or by switching the drive gas from oxygen to compressed air in a GE machine (typically done by a service technician, not an anesthesia provider or anesthesia tech).6
- CO_2 absorbent is utilized faster at low FGF and much less at high FGF. If there is a shortage of CO_2 absorbent, "...(and the supply of oxygen is not a concern): Increase total fresh gas flow to meet or exceed minute ventilation. CO_2 absorbents will be utilized very little, if at all since the goal is to reduce rebreathing. If inspired CO_2 is present on the capnogram, increasing total fresh gas flow until the inspired CO_2 is zero will eliminate rebreathing. The lack of humidity in the fresh gas may become a problem."6

Infection control

While a complete discussion is beyond the scope of this article, a few points may be made.

Protect the machine and the patient with high-efficiency HMEF at the Y piece of the breathing circuit, and at the machine end of the expiratory limb. Airway gas sampling should be done from a port on the machine side of the HMEF at the Y.

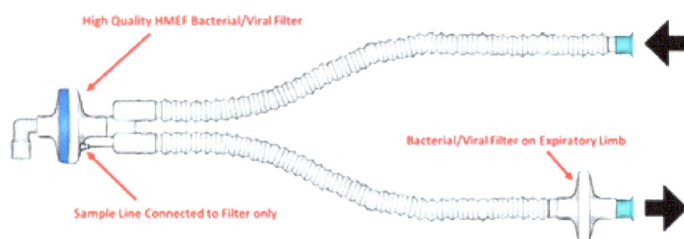

- "If the sampled gases end up in the scavenging system, no further filtering is needed."8

- "If you are using a gas analyzer that is not integrated into the anesthesia machine it is easy to trace the exhaust gas and it should go to an active (not passive) scavenging system, not the room. For integrated gas analyzers, the connections are usually hidden."8

- "If sampled gases are returned to the breathing circuit they need to be filtered [e.g. Aisys CS2 software version 11, Apollo, Perseus]. Water traps do have built-in filters and the viral filtration efficiency (VFE) determines the effectiveness.

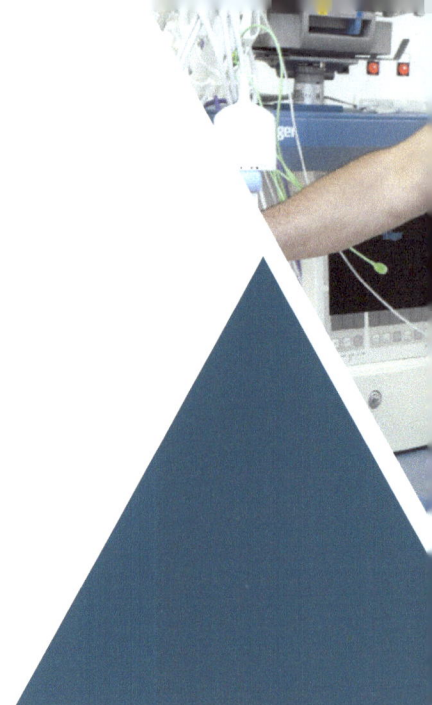

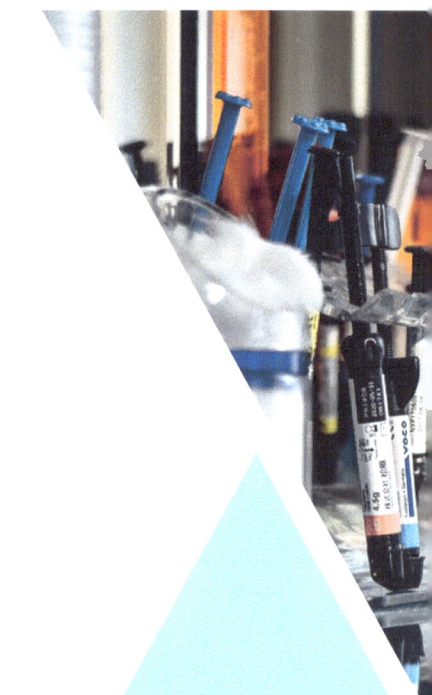

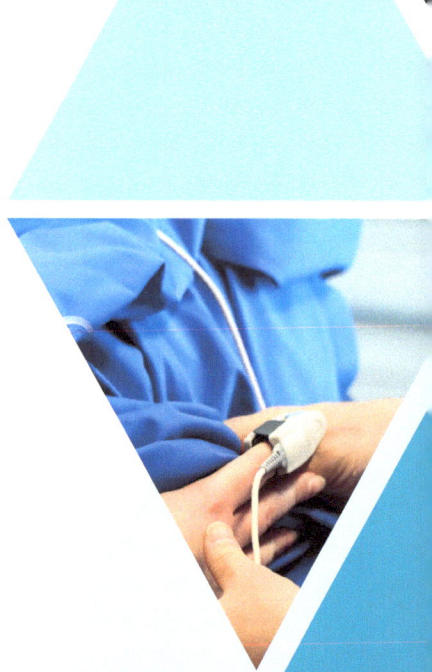

The GE DFend Pro water traps include a 0.2-micron filter with a VFE of 99.999%. Draeger uses a 0.2 micron filter in the water trap but the VFE has yet to be determined. If an airway filter option is not available, and the water trap filter cannot be confirmed, a 0.2-micron drug injection filter similar to that used in epidural kits can be placed at the water trap."8

- "If the sampled gas is routed to the scavenging system, additional filtration may not be necessary as there are standards for managing biohazards in the central suction system or waste anesthetic gas system (WAGS). Check with the local facilities manager to confirm the risk of biohazard in the suction system. Unfiltered Sampled gas should not be exhausted directly into the OR [or ICU] environment or a passive scavenging system."8

Backup

- An anesthesia workstation must never be used without a means of backup ventilation (Bag-valve-mask device [Ambu]), and an emergency cylinder supply of oxygen.

Monitoring

Continuous monitoring of airway gas (particularly inspired oxygen & capnometry), airway pressures, and volumes (tidal and minute) are absolutely essential because of the unique aspects of the anesthesia breathing circuit (rebreathing, CO_2 absorbent, scavenging, & the divergence of dialed and inspired oxygen at low FGF).1,2,6

- Alarms must be set to appropriate limits, with audible alarm volume at 100%.
- "Real-time **spirometry** (Flow-Volume and Pressure-Volume loops) is quite useful when caring for patients with respiratory failure, and for diagnosing leaks around the endotracheal tube and increased resistance through the airway HMEF."6

Periodic checks

Manufacturers highly recommend that the device be rebooted/restarted at least every 24 hours.1–3 Failing to do so results in degradation of pressure flow and volume monitoring, and breath triggering (GE), and flow measurement (but not respiratory gas monitoring -Drager). Anesthesia workstations cannot be checked while in operation, so the patient must be ventilated via alternate techniques during the 5-10 minutes required for checkout or restart.

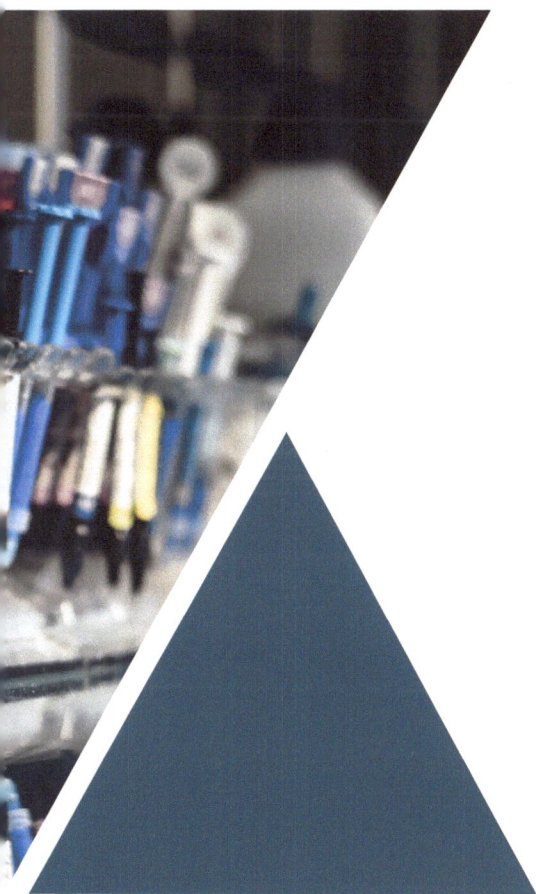

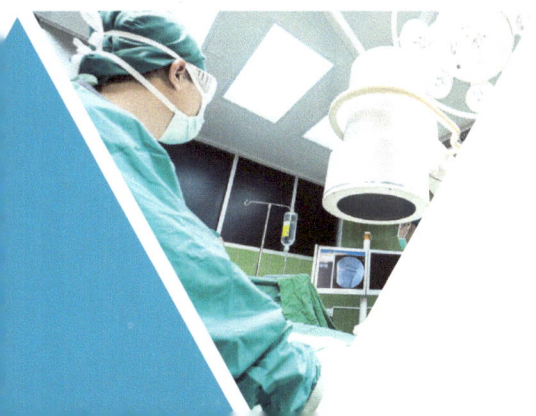

Ventilation for ARDS related to COVID-19

Most patients in normal times do not have a severe degree of lung pathology. Discussion of ventilation for ARDS is well beyond the scope of this document; Key points of that discussion are summarized below.

Anesthesia workstations are not recommended for:
long-term ventilation of pediatric or neonatal patients,1 non-invasive ventilation,1 administering nebulized drugs,2 or for ventilating multiple patients simultaneously.10

OR or ICU?

- "If the device is moved ...outside of its normal location in the OR, the device must be re-installed/configured by professionals trained in the proper setup of facility connections such as scavenging and gas inputs."1

- **"ICURooms:** At a minimum, the room requires space to accommodate the machine and sources of high-pressure air and oxygen. Scavenging is not required or necessary if appropriate viral filters are placed on the circuits. Suction outlets are available in the ICU but cannot be attached to the WAGD[waste gas] connection on the machine due to connector incompatibility."6

- "Operating Rooms: These rooms should be available in the absence of elective surgery and are appealing as isolation rooms especially if negative pressure capability is present. The anesthesia machines will be readily available for use and connected to gas supplies as well as networked for recording data to the EMR. ORs may be the only option if the ICUs become filled but have patient care drawbacks. Alarms will not be audible outside of the operating room and will need to be set to maximum volume. A caregiver will need to be continuously present in the room with the doors closed and it may be challenging to reproduce all of the ICU care resources in that location."6

"PACU beds and other hospital rooms:

PACUs are typically open with increased noise levels and the potential to spread infectious agents. Other hospital rooms may be more desirable.

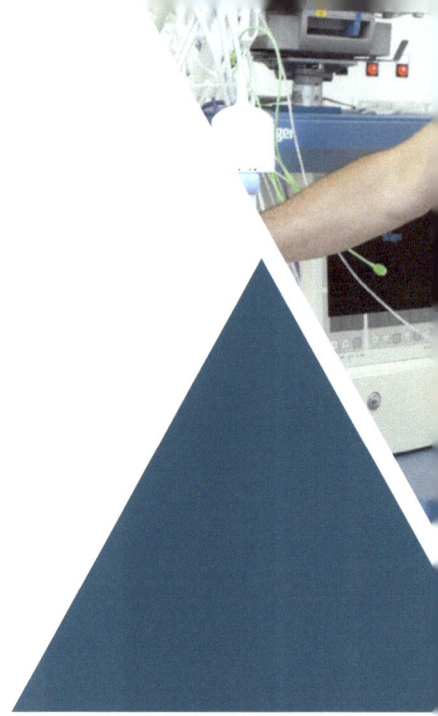

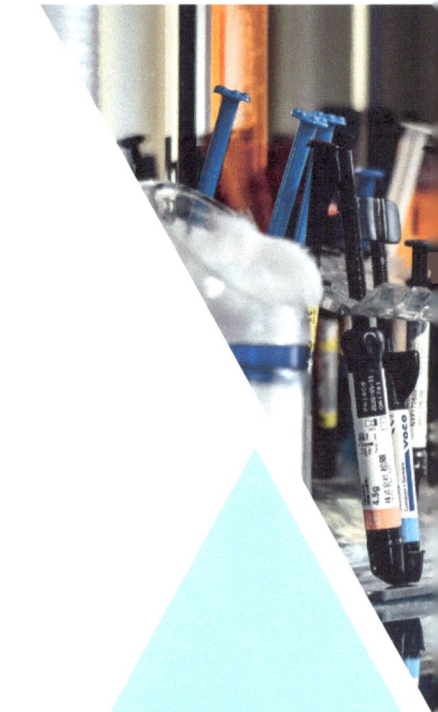

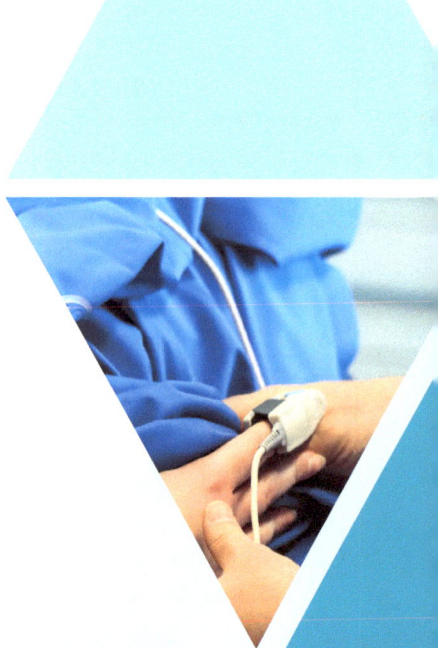

Physical space and sources of high-pressure air and oxygen are the only requirements for using the anesthesia machine as a ventilator. Wherever these machines are deployed, there will need to be an anesthesia professional immediately available and following a monitoring, schedule to ensure safe use."[6]

Settings & Targets

Mode - either pressure or volume control is acceptable.[9]

Tidal volume (VT): For lung protective ventilation, the suggested starting VT is 6 mL/kg ideal body weight (range 4-8).[9] Ideal body weight is also known as predicted body weight (PBW). Some electronic medical records calculate and display ideal BW. If you need to calculate it, see Clinical Mathematics for Anesthetists.[11]

- -   For the average **US female** (height 5 ft 4 in), starting VT is 330 mL (range 220-440). Over heights from 60-72 in, starting VT is 270-440 mL/kg.

- -   For the average **US male** (height 5 ft 9 in), stating VT is 425 mL (range 280-560). Overweight from 60-72 in, starting VT is 300-460 mL/kg.

FIO2 & PEEP-

- "...set PEEP at 5 cm H2O and FIO2 at 1 at the onset of initiation of mechanical ventilation; the FIO2 is rapidly weaned over the next hour to target a peripheral saturation (SpO2) of 88 to 95 percent (typically low to mid-90s)."[9] Keep in mind that FIO2 of 1.0 promotes atelectasis through absorption of all the oxygen in poorly-ventilated alveoli. Keeping some nitrogen in the breathing mixture (FIO2 0.8 or less) prevents atelectasis from this cause.[12]

Respiratory rate (RR)-

- "... initial VT is set at 6 mL/kg Predicted Body Weight and the initial respiratory rate is set to meet the patient's minute ventilation requirements, provided it is <35 breaths per minute (most often between 14 and 22 breaths/minute). "[9]

SpO2-

- the target is peripheral saturation (SpO2) of 88 to 95 percent (typically low to mid-90s)."[9]

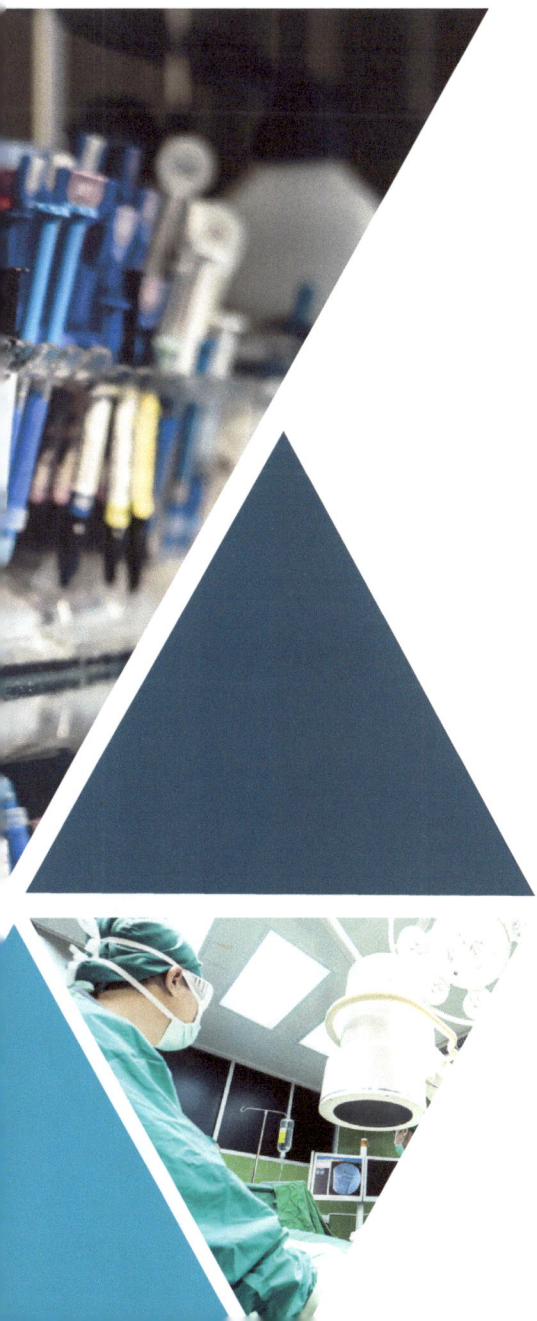

pETCO2 & Permissive hypercapnia –

- "Hypercapnic respiratory acidosis ... is an expected and generally well-tolerated consequence of LTVV [Low TidalVolume Ventiltion]. LTVV may require permissive hypercapnic ventilation, a strategy that accepts alveolar hypoventilation in order to maintain a low alveolar pressure and minimize the complications of alveolar overdistension (eg, ventilator-associated lung injury). The degree of hypercapnia can be minimized by using the highest respiratory rate that does not induce auto-PEEP."9

Plateau pressure (Pplat)-

Pplat can be measured directly if volume control with inspiratory pause is utilized. "Over the next one to four hours, the patient's clinical response, gas exchange, and Pplat can be used to adjust the VT and respiratory rate, if necessary. Clinicians are encouraged to make bedside adjustments to VT to ensure lung protective ventilation is being appropriately administered and to assess response in real-time before obtaining arterial blood gases. Typically adjustments are made simultaneously to meet clinical and gas exchange, as well as Pplat parameters...
The goal Pplat **is ≤30 cm H2O..."9**

- "When the Pplat is>30 cm H2O and the VT is set at 6 mL/kg PBW or higher, the VT should be decreased in 1 mL/kg PBW increments to a minimum of 4 mL/kg PBW to reach the target plateau. Importantly, any decrease in VT may need to
- be accompanied by an increase in respiratory rate to maintain an acceptable minute ventilation."9

Driving pressure-

Lung-protective ventilation strategies are associated with limited driving pressure ... we track driving pressure in patients in severe or refractory ARDS to identify those with recruitable lungs who may benefit from high levels of PEEP. Although a cutoff value has not been agreed upon, we and others use a target ... **< 20 mmHg.**"9 Driving pressure may be calculated as:
- -   ventilator-measured Pplat minus applied PEEP, or -   VT /respiratory system compliance, or
- -   (modified as) Peak inspiratory pressure minus PEEP.

Alveolar recruitment maneuvers (ARM)-

- Open lung strategies include ARM, which "... recruit additional atelectatic alveolar units and the applied PEEP maintains alveolar recruitment and minimizes cyclic atelectasis; this combination,in theory, should reduce the risk of inducing further lung injury by the mechanical ventilator itself."9 There is no consensus on one way to perform an ARM.

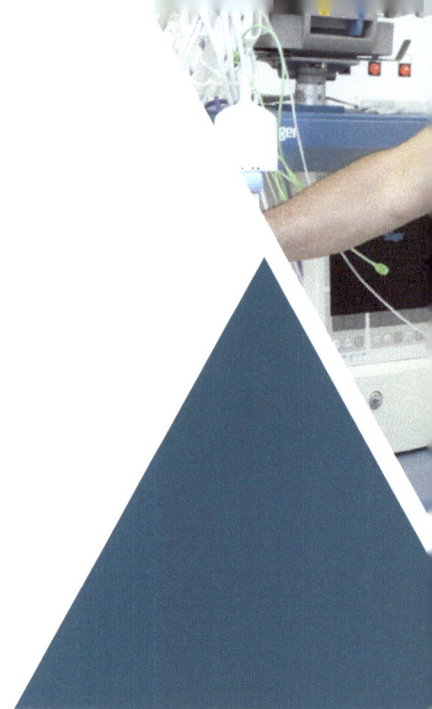

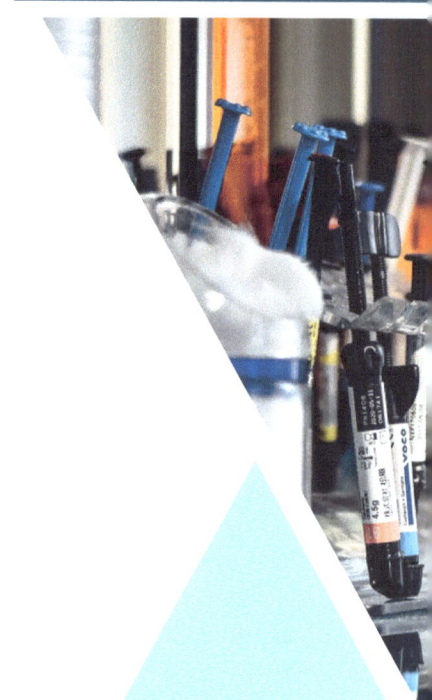

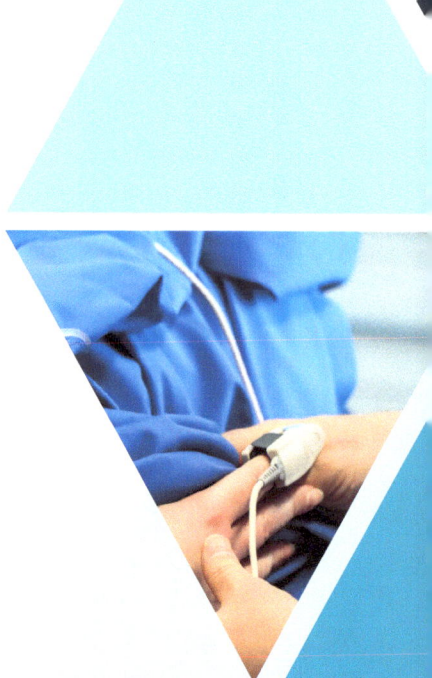

The Aisys has two strategies built in (under the Procedures [1] button on the main screen)- one which holds a selectable pressure (try 30 cmH2O) for a selectable time (try 15-20 seconds). Monitor blood pressure, because increasing mean intrathoracic pressure can decrease venous return.

pH -

"There is no consensus regarding an acceptable lower or upper limit for pH ... most experts agree that ... a pH below 7.25 and above 7.5 should be addressed while maintaining LTVV (ie, a VT between 4 and 8 mL/kg PBW and a pPlat ≤30 cm H2O)."[9]

Alternative means of ventilation -

If resources are ultimately strained, last-ditch alternatives to consider might include Simple devices operating in volume control (Bear) or pressure control mode (Bird), or manual ventilation by the Bag-valve-mask device.[13–15]

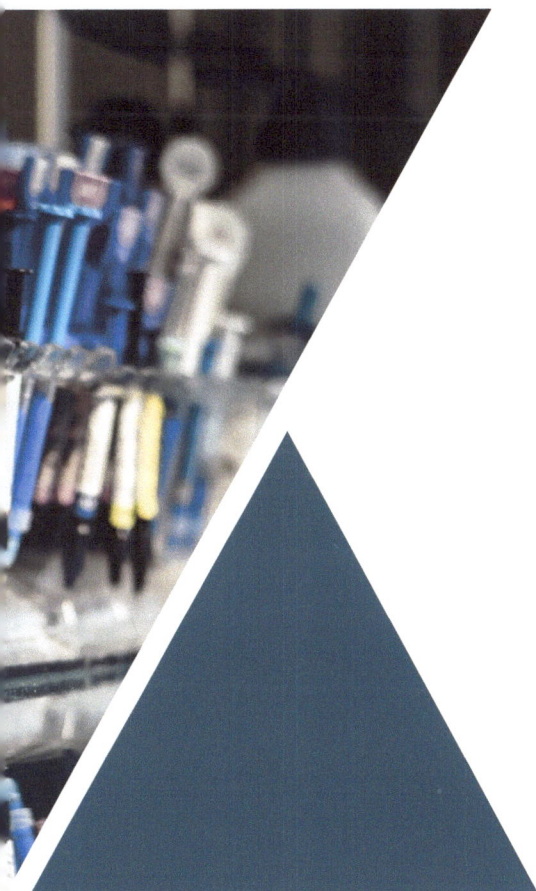

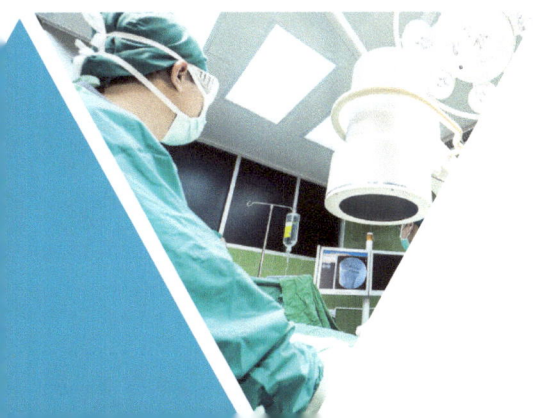

References

1.   GE Healthcare. Topic: COVID-19 - Requests for information regarding the off-label use of GE Healthcare anesthesia devices for ICU ventilation. https://www.gehealthcare.com/-/jssmedia/3c655c83bd6b427e9824994c12be0da5.pdf?la=en-us. Accessed March 29, 2020.

2.   Thams I, Heesch R, Rahlf-Luong M. COVID-19: Usage of Dräger anaesthesia devices for long-term ventilation. https://www.draeger.com/Library/Content/Draeger Customer Letter - COVID-19 -Usage of Anesthesia devices for long-term ventilation-2020-03-18.pdf. Accessed March 29, 2020.

3.   Arpino D.Mindray A-Series Anesthesia Delivery System Consideration for use as a Ventilator March 23, 2020. https://www.mindraynorthamerica.com/wp-content/uploads/2020/03/1658B-Considerations-for-MR-Anes-Sys-used-for-Ventilators-during-COVID-19-1.pdf. Accessed March 29, 2020.

4.   US Food and Drug Administration. Ventilator Supply Mitigation Strategies: Letter to Health Care Providers 3-22-20. https://www.fda.gov/medical-devices/letters-health-care-providers/ventilator-supply-mitigation-strategies-letter-health-care-providers. Accessed March 29, 2020.

5.   Coronavirus (COVID-19) Update: FDA takes action to help increase U.S. supply of ventilators and respirators for protection of health care workers, patients. March 27, 2020. https://www.fda.gov/news-events/press-announcements/coronavirus-covid-19-update-fda-takes-action-help-increase-us-supply-ventilators-and-respirators. Accessed March 31, 2020.

6.   American Society of Anesthesiologists, Anesthesia Patient Safety Foundation. APSF/ASA Guidance on Purposing Anesthesia Machines as ICU Ventilators. https://www.asahq.org/in-the-spotlight/coronavirus-covid-19-information/purposing-anesthesia-machines-for-ventilators. Accessed March 29, 2020.

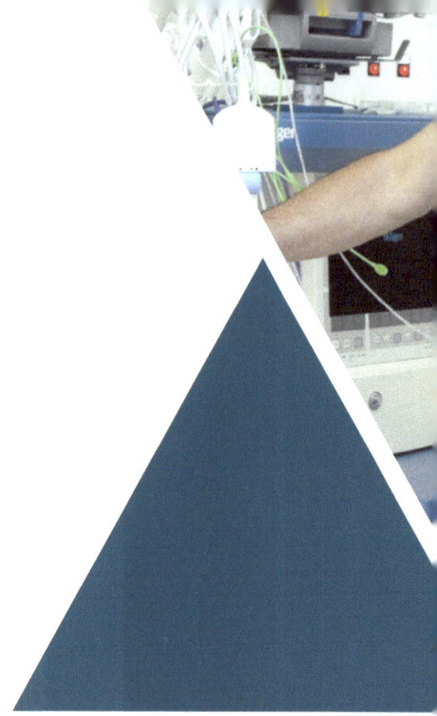

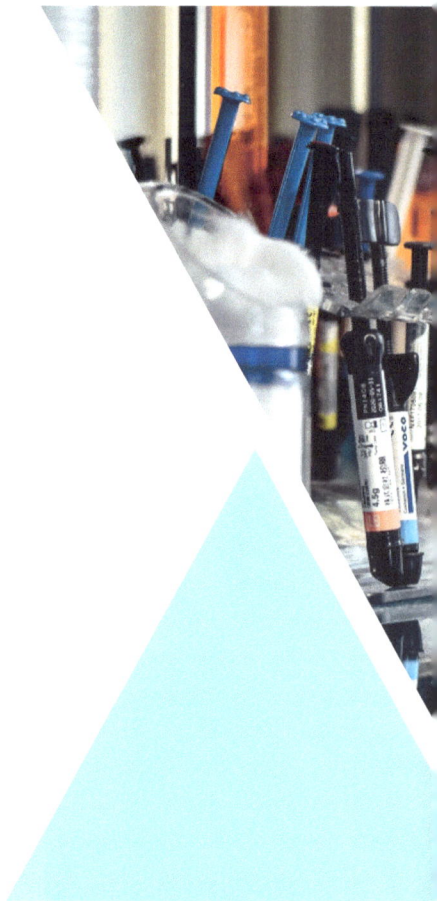

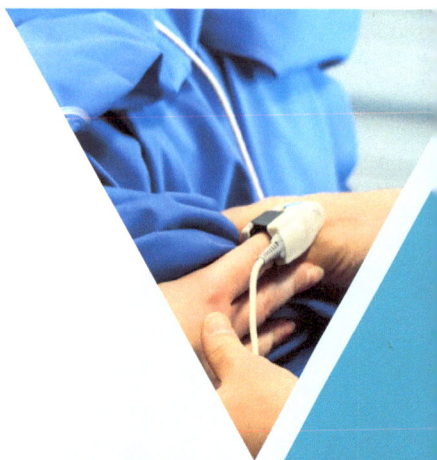

7.   Thal S,Martensen A. SARS-CoV-2 and handling of Dräger Anesthesia Workstations, February 20, 2020. https://www.draeger.com/Library/Content/SARS-CoV-2-and-handling-of-Draeger-Anesthesia-Workstations.pdf. Accessed March 29, 2020.

8.   Feldman J, Loeb R, Philip J. FAQ on Anesthesia Machine use, protection, and decontamination during the COVID-19 pandemic. https://www.apsf.org/faq-on-anesthesia-machine-use-protection-and-decontamination-during-the-covid-19-pandemic/. Accessed March 29, 2020.

9.   Siegel M,Hyzy R. Ventilator management strategies for adults with acute respiratory distress syndrome. Up to Date. https://www.uptodate.com/contents/ventilator-management-strategies-for-adults-with-acute-respiratory-distress-syndrome. Accessed March 29, 2020.

10.   Anesthesia Patient Safety Foundation. Joint Statement on Multiple Patients Per Ventilator. https://www.apsf.org/news-updates/joint-statement-on-multiple-patients-per-ventilator/. Accessed March 29, 2020.

11.   Dosch M. Clinical Mathematics for Anesthetists. https://healthprofessions.udmercy.edu/academics/na/agm/mathweb09.pdf. AccessedMarch 30, 2020.

12.   Weenink RP, de Jonge SW,Preckel B, Hollmann MW. Use 80% oxygen not only during extubation but throughout anesthesia. Anesth Analg. 2020;130(3):e96-e97. doi:10.1213/ANE.0000000000004587

13.   Halpern P, Dang T, Epstein Y, Van Stijn-Bringas D, Koenig K. Six hours of manual ventilation with a Bag-valve-mask device is feasible and clinically consistent. Crit CareMed. 2019;47:e222. doi:10.1097/CCM.0000000000003632.

14.   Stoddart J. Some observations on the function of the Bird Mark 8 ventilator. Br J Anaesth. 1966;38:977. doi:10.1093/bja/38.12.977

15.   KacmarekR. The Mechanical Ventilator: Past, Present, and Future. Respir Care. 2011;56:1170-1180. doi:10.4187/respcare.01420

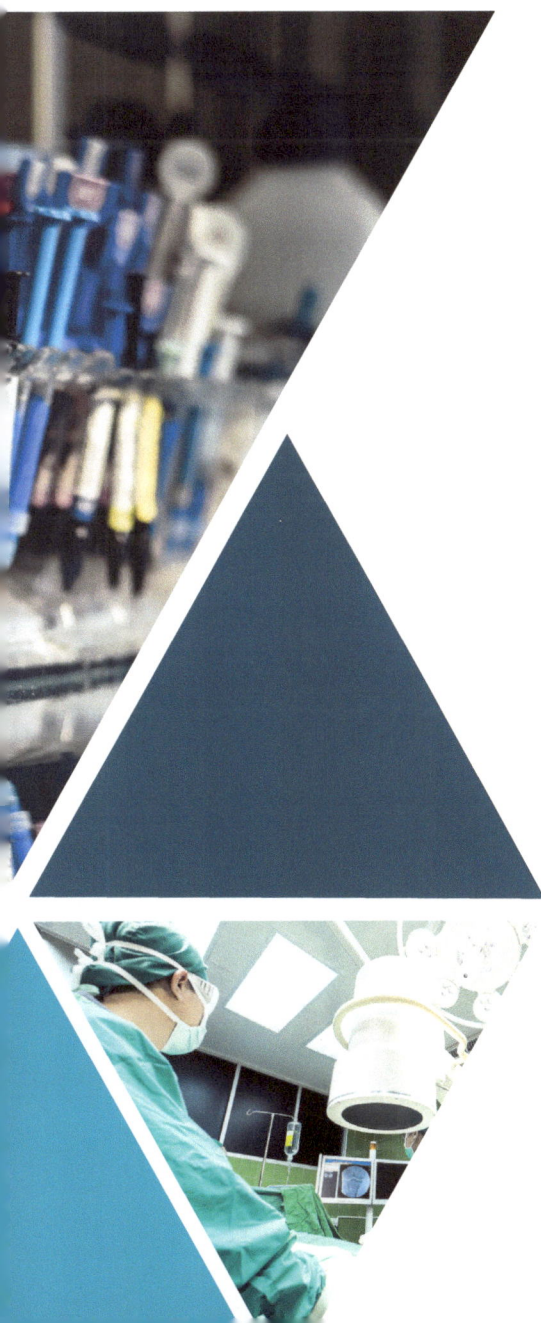

Disclosures, Disclaimer,and Acknowledgements

Use of the anesthesia workstation as a ventilator for critically ill patients is an off-label use of the device, is entirely the responsibility of the user, and should be carefully considered before implementation. Any recommendations herein should be subject to local anesthesia provider before implementation.

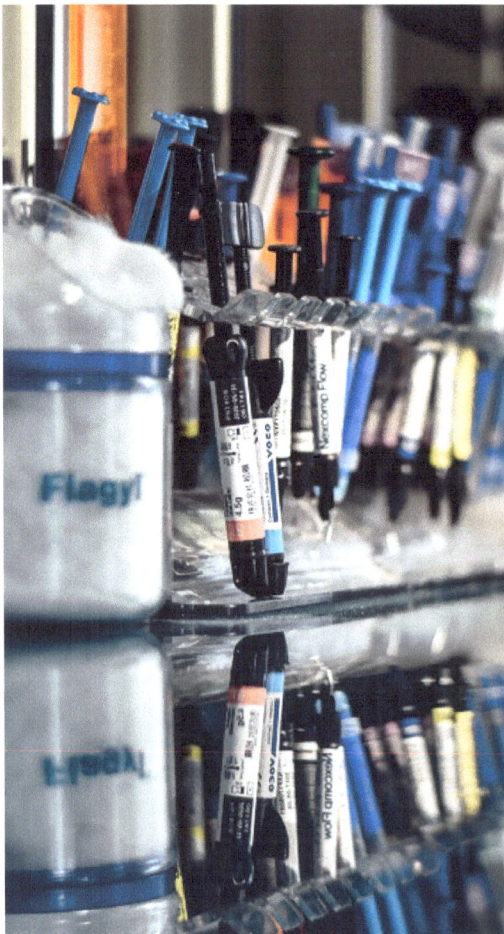

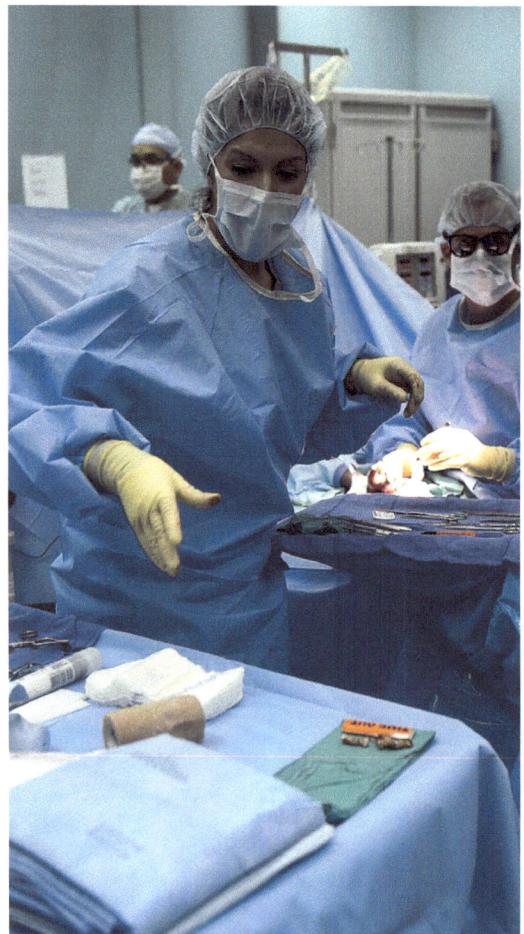

Anesthesia for Thoracic Surgical Procedures

Introduction

As thoracic surgery evolved, and anesthesia evolved in parallel, allowing even the most complicated surgical procedures to be performed relatively safely. This co-evolution mirrors the close association of the thoracic surgeon and anesthesiologist when caring for their patients. Thisuniqueassociation is predicated on the nature of thoracic procedures, where the surgeon and anesthesiologist share a "thoracic workspace" - the surgeon operating on vital thoracic structures and the anesthesiologist managing ventilation, oxygenation, and hemodynamics. Because of this close partnering, it is valuable for thoracic surgeons to be familiar with aesthetic considerations, exclusive to their patients.

2. Considerationsfor One-Lung Ventilation (OLV)

Thoracic Surgery poses unique challenges to the anesthesiologist, including surgery in the lateral decubitus position, an open thorax, manipulation of thoracic organs, potential for major bleeding, and, unique among all potential surgery scenarios, the need for lung isolation.

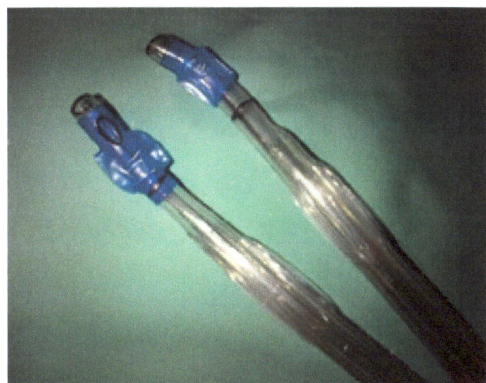

2.1. Physiologic effects of lung isolation

Successful lung isolation (one-lung ventilation, OLV) requires the management of oxygenation, ventilation, and pulmonary blood flow. Remarkably, OLV decreases total minute ventilation minimally. In fact, it has been shown that the non-isolated lung receives close to the same minute of ventilation as ventilation to two lungs. The rate of CO_2 elimination undergoes minimal changes because CO_2 is readily diffusible and has no plateau in its dissociation curve

When a patient is placed on OLV, inevitably a shunt is developed. The non-dependent lung is no longer being ventilated but is still perfused, resulting in a right to left shunt. When this occurs, the pulmonary system has physiological adaptations to decrease this shunt. Given that the patient is in the lateral decubitus position, one of the responses is a decrease in blood flow to the non-dependent lung due to gravitational forces. These effects are significant because the pulmonary system has a much lower blood pressure than the systemic circulation.

Another adaptation is hypoxic pulmonary vasoconstriction of the vascular supply in the non-dependent lung. Hypoxic pulmonary vasoconstriction is a physiological phenomenon in which pulmonary arteries constrict in the presence of hypoxia (unlike the systemic circulation), redirecting blood flow to the dependent lung. Surgical compression of the non-dependent lung can also serve as a way of decreasing shunt as the pulmonary vasculature is compressed. One last factor contributing to a decrease in shunt fraction is apneic oxygenation—residual oxygen in the non-dependent isolated lung diffusing into the pulmonary circulation. All these factors combined allow for better oxygenation during OLV.

2.2. Preoperative anesthetic evaluation of the thoracic surgery patient

Patients undergoing OLV should undergo a perioperative assessment of their respiratory function that includes testing of lung mechanical function, pulmonary parenchymal function, and cardiopulmonary reserve. The best assessment of respiratory function comes from a history of the patient's quality of life. It is useful to think of respiratory function in three related but independent areas: respiratory mechanics, gas exchange, and cardio-respiratory interaction.

Themostvalidtestforperioperativeassessmentofrespiratorymechanicsisthepredictedpost-operative forced expiratory volume in one second(ppoFEV1). This test is the best at predicting post-thoracotomy respiratory complications.

Percentage of predicted postoperative (ppo) FEV1 after lobectomy is given by

ppoFEV1= preoperative FEV1 x No. of segments remaining

Nakahara et al found that patients with a ppoFEV1 of more than 40% had no or only minor post-resection respiratory complications. Major respiratory complications were only seen in the sub-group with ppoFEV1 < 40%; post-operative mechanical ventilator support was seen in those<30%.

For the assessment of lung parenchymal function, the most useful test of the gas exchange capacity is the diffusing capacity for carbon monoxide (DLCO). This test correlates with the total functioning surface of the alveolar-capillary interface. The DLCO is used to calculate a post-resection value using the same calculation as FEV1. A ppoDLCO less than 40% of predicted correlates with increased cardiac and respiratory complications and is relatively independent of the FEV1.

Stairclimbingisthemosttraditionaltestofrespiratoryfunctionintheassessmentofcardiopulmonaryinteraction. Ability to climb three flights or more is closely associated with a decrease in morbidity and mortality. The ability to climb fewer than two flights is associated with a very high risk. The "gold standard" for assessment is formal laboratory exercise testing with maximal oxygen consumption. Climbing five flights of stairs approximates a VO2 max value of >20 ml/kg/min and less than one flight is associated with values <10 ml/kg/ min (S9). Ventilation-perfusion (V/Q) scintigraphy can also be used as a preoperative assessment when pulmonary resection is to be undertaken.

Thismodalityisparticularlyhelpfulfor patients undergoing pneumonectomy or any patient with a ppoFEV1 less than 40%.

Slinger et al. proposed a "3-legged" stool of pre-thoracotomy respiratory assessment, which encompasses the prior mentioned pre-operative tests. This model summarizes the results of those tests and reveals that patients have lower expected post-operative morbidity if they have a ppoFEV1 > 40%, cardio-pulmonary reserve with a VO2 max >15 ml/kg/min, and lung parenchymal function with a ppoDLCO >40%.

These three tests are the most valid for pre-operative assessment. Other tests that can be used are maximal volume ventilation(MVV), residual volume/total lung capacity (RV/TLC), and forced vital capacity (FVC), but these are less valid for respiratory mechanics. Stair climbing (two flights), a 6-minute walk, and measurement in the change in SpO2 (<4%) during exercise are other tests that can be used to measure cardiopulmonary reserve. Measurement of arterial blood gas values can also serve. as a respiratory assessment; indicators of good prognosisarePaO2 > 60 and a PaCO2 < 45.

In regards to post-thoracotomy anesthetic management, Slinger et al. devised an algorithm derived from a pre-operative assessment using ppoFEV1. If the patient's ppoFEV1 is > 40%and the patient is awake, alert, warm, and comfortable, immediate postoperative extubation is recommended. If the ppoFEV1 is between 30-40%, extubation should be considered based on exercise tolerance, DLCO, V/Q scan, and associated diseases. If the ppoFEV1 < 30%, stage weaning from mechanical ventilation is recommended. However, when the patient has a functioning thoracic epidural catheter providing adequate analgesia, extubation may beattempted even at ppoFEV1values as low as20%.

2.3. Tracheo-bronchial anatomy for lung isolation

Knowledge of tracheo-bronchial anatomy is important for achieving and maintaining proper lung isolation. Other chapters in this text describe lung and bronchial anatomy in detail. Features of the anatomy that are relevant to anesthetic considerations are presented here

Acriticall and mark when placing lung isolation devices is the primary carina, where the trachea splits into two main bronchi. The diversion angle differs between these main bronchi, with the right bronchi angled at 25 degrees and the left bronchus at 45 degrees. Because of the steeper angle of diversion of the right main bronchus, foreign bodies (including lung isolation devices) are more likely to travel into this bronchus. Left and right-side double lumen tubes(DLTs)are designed with curvatures to accommodate left or right main bronchi diversion angles to make intubation into the specified main bronchi easier(Figure 1).

Because of the steeper angle of the right mainstem bronchus, it is not uncommon to inadvertently intubate the right mainstem when intending to intubate the left mainstem with a DLT (using blind or non-fiber optic guided placement techniques). Operators unfamiliar with distal bronchial anatomy sometimes confuse secondary carinas with the primary carina. For example, the right main bronchus divides at the secondary carina into the upper lobar bronchus and bronchus intermedius; this secondary carina may be mistaken for the primary carina when viewed under bronchoscopy. Therefore, knowledge of distal bronchial anatomy is fundamental in confirming correct placement as well as in correcting misplacement.

Knowledge of distal bronchial anatomy is essential for additional reasons. First, the operator must recognize that a right DLT has an additional slot to allow for ventilation of the right upper lobe and must place it at the correct depth and rotational alignment to assure adequate ventilation of all three lobes. Secondly, anatomy is abnormal in a small percentage of patients. For example, in up to 2% of patients, the right bronchus originates directly from the supra carinal trachea (a so-called bronchus suis). Abnormal anatomy is also seen in patients who have had previous lung surgeries. The operator must be able to recognize and respond to abnormal anatomy by selecting the appropriate device to provide effect lung isolation inany scenario.

2.4. Indications for lung isolation

Patient pathology and/or operative requirements determine the indication for OLV. Patients with lung pathology may need lung protection. For example, OLV may be used to protect the affected lung from contamination with pus or blood from the affected lung. Alternatively, OLV may be used to provide differential lung ventilation to minimize volutrauma and barotrauma to the affected lung while optimizing ventilation to the non-affected lung. Certainoperative scenarios require OLV. Because it optimizes visualization of the operative site, OLVis absolutely indicated in closed procedures (for example, thoracoscopic surgery) but is also useful in open procedures to maximize exposure.

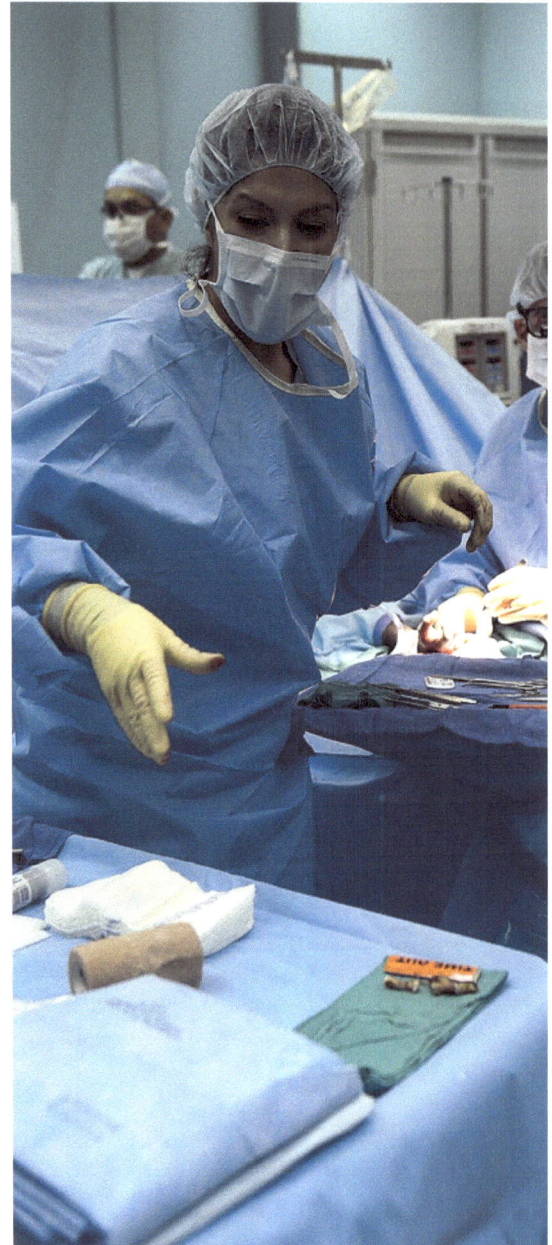

2.5. Lung isolation devices

Three standard methods for lung isolation include DLT, bronchial blockers, and mainstem intubation.

2.5.1. DLT

The standard device for providing lung isolation is the DLT. It provides reliable lung isolation, offers the ability to suction both lungs, allows for bilateral differential lung ventilation with minimal device manipulation, and allows for simple procedures such as broncho alveolar lavage. DLTs range in size from 28 to 41 Fr. Posteroanterior (PA) chest x-ray is the standard method of sizing comparison between DLT, trachea, and bronchial diameter. However, patient sex, age, and height are commonly used to choose DLT size. As discussed above, DLTsaremade in right-side and left-side conformations to accommodate the differences in the anatomy of the right and left main bronchi (i.e., the right upper lobe branch).

2.5.2. SLT with bronchial blocker

Bronchial blockers used with conventional single lumen tubes have advantages in difficult airways, in patients with indwelling endotracheal or tracheostomy tubes, in patients who are nasally intubated with SLTs, and in cases where sub-segmental blockade may be required. Bronchial blockers have several disadvantages, however. They are easier to displace and provide limited suction and drainage to the isolated lung, which may lead to an accumulation of pus, blood, or secretions. They are deployed in the operative lung, which may interfere with the surgical procedure, and the device must be repositioned for contralateral lung isolation.

Despite their specific enhancements, bronchial blockers are essentially modeled after vascular embolization catheters (albeit with high compliance low-pressure cuffs, and a deflation port).

They are manufactured as separate units or units integrated with an endotracheal tube. Separate units include the Cohen Flexi-tip BB (Cook Critical Care), Fuji Uni-blocker (FujiSystems, Tokyo) (Figure 2A), and the Arndt wire-guided BB (Cook Critical Care, Bloomington, IN) (Figure2B). An example of an integrated unit is the Univent tube (Fuji Systems, Tokyo).

2.5.3. Mainstem intubation

Mainstem bronchial intubation with an SLT may be used for lung isolation in emergent scenarios or in pediatric cases. However, with this method, exhalation of the operative lung is limited, airway protection at the vocal cords is compromised, and the endotracheal tube tip is advanced into the operative lung; lastly, repositioning is required if contralateral isolation is needed. Furthermore, standard endotracheal tubes may be too short to effectively mainstem intubate either main bronchi; specialized longer tubes, such as Micro Laryngoscopy Tubes (MLTs), may be required.

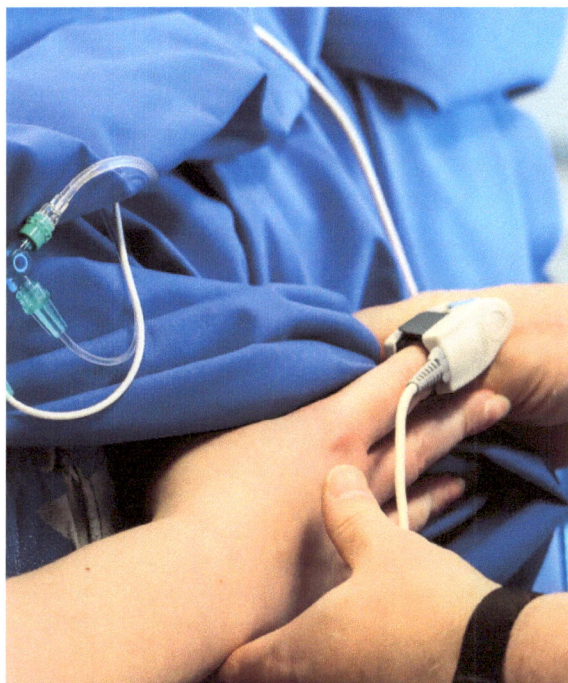

2.6. Difficult airway and lung isolation

Campos describes two categories of patients at risk for difficult intubation during OLV: those with complications related to the upper airway and those related to the lower airway. The former includes a short neck and increased neck circumference, prominent upper incisors with a receding mandible, limited cervical mobility, limited jaw opening due to previous surgery, radiation therapy of the neck, previous hemiglossectomy, or hemi mandibulectomy, and tumors of the upper airway.

Lower airway risk factors include an existing tracheotomy, a distorted tracheobronchial anatomy, and compression at the entrance of the left mainstem bronchus. Patients with any of the above conditions might pose a difficulty for lung isolation with a conventional DLT and might be candidates for SLT placement with subsequent lung isolation with a bronchial blocker. However, if a DLT is indicated, fiberoptic intubation may be used to facilitate placement. However, because of the long length of the DLT, it is difficult to maintain distal control of the fiberscope, especially with patients having longer or alto vocal cord distance. Additionally, the small diameter bronchoscope required (to assure fit for the DLT) results in an inferior view and restricts suction capabilities.

(a)

(b)

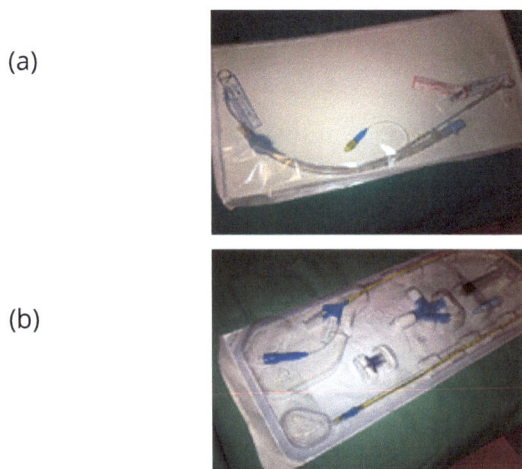

Figure 2. Examples of bronchial blockers. (A) Fuji Uni-blocker (Fuji Systems, Tokyo); (B) Arndt wire-guided BB (Cook Critical Care, Bloomington, IN)

Therefore, new generation indirect laryngoscopes may be preferable. Indirect laryngoscopes (e.g., CMAC[Storz, Tuttlingen, Germany], GlideScope [Verathon, Bothell, WA], Airtraq (Prodol Meditec S.A., Vizcaya, Spain)) improve airway grade and have been shown to improve the ease of intubation with DLTs in patients with difficult airways.

2.7. Confirming proper lung isolation

Regardless of the device used for lung isolation, the anesthesiologist must confirm correct placement of the device. Chest auscultation has traditionally been used to confirm correct DLTplacement. The process is straightforward in patients with normal pulmonary anatomy.
First, inflate both tracheal and bronchial balloons and auscultate to confirm bilateral breath sounds(if bilateral breath sounds are absent, suspect malposition– the DLT may be too deep). Next, sequentially clamp the tracheal and bronchial inflow limbs of the DLT and auscultate the chest. Absent breath sounds corresponding to the tracheal or bronchial lumen clamped, should be confirmed.

Different malposition scenarios may be deduced depending on the type of DLT (L v. R), intended mainstem to be intubated, DLT lumen occluded, and the absence or presence of breath sounds. Although auscultation is an important tool in situations where fiberoptic bronchoscopy is unavailable, studies have shown a large margin of positioning error when it is not used [15-18]. Fiberopticconfirmation is required for proper positioning of bronchial blockers because they lack basic ergonomic design features that enable blind placement (like curvature or specialized ventilation port configurations of DLTs). Furthermore, because a positioned lung isolation devices may be potentially be fatal, and auscultation is usually not an option intraoperatively, fiberoptic bronchoscopy has become the standard for proper placement and maintenance of lung isolation devices.

3. Intraoperativecare for the thoracic surgical patient

3.1. Ventilator strategies for one-lung ventilation

For thoracic surgery, the incidence of pulmonary complications now out-numbers that of cardiovascular complications, and pulmonary complications are the most common cause of postoperative death in esophageal cancer patients.

Injury from one-lung ventilation(OLV)can manifest as re-expansion pulmonary edema (REPE), acute lung injury (ALI), or acute respiratory distress syndrome (ARDS). While late causes of ALI (3-10 days after surgery)are secondary to bronchopneumonia or aspiration, early ALI is predicted by high intraoperative ventilation pressures, increased surgery duration, excessive intravenous volume replacement, pneumonectomy, and preoperative alcohol abuse.

Most likely, a combination of a patient's health status, intraoperative fluid management, the use of epidural analgesia, inflammatory responses due to surgical manipulation, alveolar recruitment, and re-expansion/reperfusion lung injury [22, 23] underlie the development of ALI following OLV. While chronic patient risk factors are difficult to modify, protective ventilatory strategies and judicious fluid use may decrease the incidence of ALI.

Prior ventilatory schemes focused on the detrimental effects of atelectasis, primarily increased pulmonary shunt via local alveolar hypoxia and hyperoxia. Tidal volumes of 10-12mL/kg were advocated, as it was previously held that tidal volumes <8mL/kg resulted in decreased functional residual capacity (FRC) and worsening atelectasis in the dependent lung.

The lowest positive end-expiratory pressure (PEEP) for acceptable oxygenation and normal arterial CO_2 levels (35to38mmHg) were suggested. OLV was achieved with parameters similar to two-lung ventilation, with consequent stimulation of stretch-activated cation channels,oxygen-derived free radicals, activated neutrophils, and cytokine upregulation contributing to increased microvascular-alveolar permeability

The current strategy to minimize OLV-associated lung injury utilizes so-called lung protective ventilation. Overdistension (volutrauma), excessive transpulmonary pressure resulting in barotrauma, repeated opening and closing of alveoli resulting in ateleto trauma, and biotrauma caused by inflammatory mediators are considered contributing factors to ventilator-induced lung injury (VILI).

These factors combined may induce inflammatory changes in pulmonary alveolar and vascular endothelium, predisposing them to pathological apoptosis and necrosis. In this way, VILI can both exacerbate existing lung injury and sensitize the lung to further injury via a two-hit model.

Reduction of tidal volumes during OLV to 5ml/kg was shown to reduce the alveolar concentration of TNF-αand sICAM-1 (will it be obvious to the reader what implications this has?). Moreover, with fixed tidal volumes of 9mL/kg, the addition of 5cm H_2O PEEP was associated with better oxygenation and earlier extubation.

PEEP improves the (ventilation: perfusion) V:Q relationship via increased FRC at end expiration. However, excessive PEEP may redistribute blood flow away from the dependent ventilated lung.

Thus, protective ventilation consists of:

- maintaining the fraction of inspiredO2 (Fi02) as low as possible to avoid absorption atelectasis and worsening shunt

- PEEP above the lower inflection point on the static pressure-volume curve
- a tidal volume of 5-6mL/kg, plateau pressures of less than 20cmH2O above the PEEP value
- peak inspiratory pressures less than 35 cm H2O
- respiratory rate(RR) 10-18
- inspiratory: expiratory (I:E) ratio1:2 to1:3
- permissive hypercapnia
- preferential use of pressure-limited ventilatory modes

Hypoxemia may require continuous positive airway pressure (CPAP) to the nondependent lung, allowing apneic oxygenation and increasing the overall partial pressure of O2 (pa02). Permissive hypercapnia is generally tolerated with protective ventilator strategies during OLV. Not only does hypocapnia worsen the parenchymal and ischemia-reperfusion injury, but hypercapnia itself may have beneficial effects on serum cytokine levels, apoptosis, and free radical injury. The optimal level of paCO2 has not been determined.

Pressure-controlled ventilation achieves lower airway pressure, and the homogeneous distribution of inspired gas allows the recruitment of collapsed lungs and improved oxygenation. This method is thought to minimize end-inspiratory distension and collapse of lung units and has demonstrated a decreased inflammatory response, improved lung function, and earlier extubation. As compared with conventional ventilation, this protective strategy was associated with improved survival at 28days, a higher rate of weaning from mechanical ventilation, and a lower rate of barotrauma in patients with ARDS. However, protective ventilation was not associated with a higher rate of survival to hospital discharge. Even with protective lung ventilatory strategies, it is possible that certain patchy segments of alveoli are intermittently and inconsistently recruited, resulting in impaired surfactant effectiveness and barotrauma.

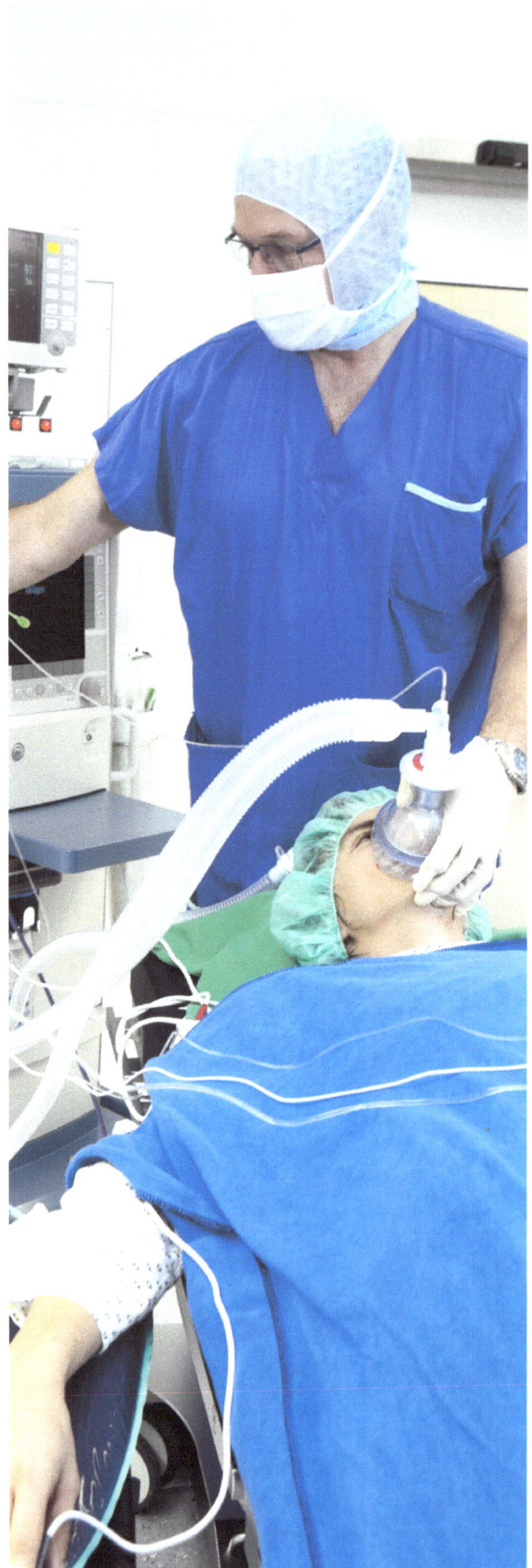

Lung protective ventilation primarily refers to the dependent lung, which shows a more pronounced inflammatory response than the nonventilated lung [33, 34]. However, it is likely that the overall postoperative clinical picture amounts to the combination of differing insults to the operative and nonoperative lung.

Hypoxia-induced lung inflammation and stress-induced mechanical injury affects the operative lung as well, as the atelectatic, nonventilated lung is periodically inflated to assess air leaks. Additionally, the operative lung is subject to pulmonary contusion due to surgical manipulation and mechanical trauma.

After 30 minutes of OLV, the collapsed lung releases inflammatory mediators into the epithelial lining fluid, indicating tissue insult and possibly resulting in systemic physiological changes . Finally, barotrauma may occur at the end of OLV as previously atelectatic alveolar units are recruited. The contribution of the type of anesthetic to the inflammatory response and clinical outcomes is currently unknown.

Studies comparing propofol to volatile anesthetics such as sevoflurane and desflurane have yielded conflicting results . Overall, differences in surgical time, duration of OLV, and laboratory techniques in existing studies have complicated interpretations of the data. Volatile agents are thought to have immune-modulating effects. While previous work showed anti-inflammatory effects of propofol, recent studies have demonstrated decreased inflammatory markers in both the operative and nonoperative lung with volatile anesthesia[36-38].

Sugasawa and colleagues found that sevoflurane use was significantly associated with a suppressed inflammatory response compared to propofol. Thus, the choice of anesthetic agent and other drugs such as ropivacaine, ketamine, thiopental, and dexmedetomidine may have anti-inflammatory effects that may be protective during lung surgery with OLV.

Further study is needed to elucidate the role of theseagents .

In conclusion, lung protective ventilator strategies which minimize Fi02, barotrauma, and volutrauma are currently being used during OLV. Optimal lung protection, however, is multifactorial and may also depend on fluid administration techniques and perioperative drug administration. Alternative lung protective strategies for experimental or rescue use, such as extracorporeal membrane oxygenation and high-frequency oscillatory ventilation are discussed elsewhere.

3.2. Fluid therapy — Goal-directed therapy for thoracic surgery

Intravenous fluids are administered perioperatively in order to optimize systemic oxygen delivery to meet metabolic demands. Cardiac preload, afterload, and contractility are frequently used as surrogate indicators of global tissue perfusion. Inadequate intravascular volume can predispose to ischemia and end-organ dysfunction.

Excessive fluid administration, on the other hand, can lead to tissue edema and compromised perfusion. In the operative setting, surgical insults may theoretically cause an inflammatory response characterized by alterations in microvascular integrity, allowing abnormal transmicrovascular fluid flux.

Due to this increase in microvascular permeability, interstitial edema may develop, which decreases O2 diffusion, resulting in hypoxic cell injury. This injury propagates a vicious cycle involving further cell death and the subsequent release of inflammatory cytokines.

In esophagectomy patients, the goal of intraoperative fluid administration is to balance perfusion pressure and oxygen delivery to vital organs including the gut mucosa, while preventing excessive fluid accumulation that may delay recovery of gastrointestinal function, impair wound, and anastomotic healing, coagulation, and cardiac and respiratory function.

Restrictive fluid regimens were thought to result in better gastrointestinal recovery time, reduced overall morbidity, improved respiratory parameters, decreased incidence of postoperative pulmonary complications, and shorter recovery periods. Conversely, fluid overload had a direct negative relationship to the function and structure of the intestinal anastomoses

The thoracic surgery population is particularly prone to pulmonary complications, which have significant implications for patient outcomes. In the setting of pulmonary resection, for example, postoperative pulmonary edema confers a high mortality risk.

Three significant risk factors include right pneumonectomy, increased perioperative intravenous fluids, and increased postoperative urine output. Patel (1992) found that fluid replacement of greaterthan3L in the 24 hours surrounding surgery was correlated with increased mortality. While pulmonary edema is associated with fluid overload, there is no clear causal relationship.

With histology compatible with ARDS, postpneumonectomy pulmonary edema occurs despite a normal PAOP, and the high protein content of edema fluid points toward low-pressure endothelial damage. Nevertheless, appropriate fluid administration may mitigate the deleterious effects of pulmonary pathology.

In conclusion, lung protective ventilator strategies which minimize Fi02, barotrauma, and volutrauma are currently being used during OLV. Optimal lung protection, however, is multifactorial and may also depend on fluid administration techniques and perioperative drug administration. Alternative lung protective strategies for experimental or rescue use, such as extracorporeal membrane oxygenation and high-frequency oscillatory ventilation are discussed elsewhere.

Traditional static cardiac preload measures such as CVP may fail to provide reliable estimations of actual preload and cardiac responses to fluid therapy. Studies on supine patients have demonstrated improved intraoperative hemodynamic stability, reduced ICU admissions, lower incidence of complications, and reduced mortality after major surgery with the use of dynamic preload indicators and goal-directed fluid therapy (GDT) [47, 48].

Commonly used monitors include esophageal Doppler monitoring and measures of arterial pulse pressure variation with respiration, such as the Lithium Dilution Cardiac Output (LiDCOplus) system and FloTrac/Vigileo.

Using an esophageal Doppler probe, Gan (2002) found that GDT in patients undergoing major elective general, urologic, or gynecologic surgery with an anticipated blood loss of greater than 500mL resulted in an earlier return of bowel function, lower incidence of postoperative nausea and vomiting, and decreased length of postoperative hospital stay.

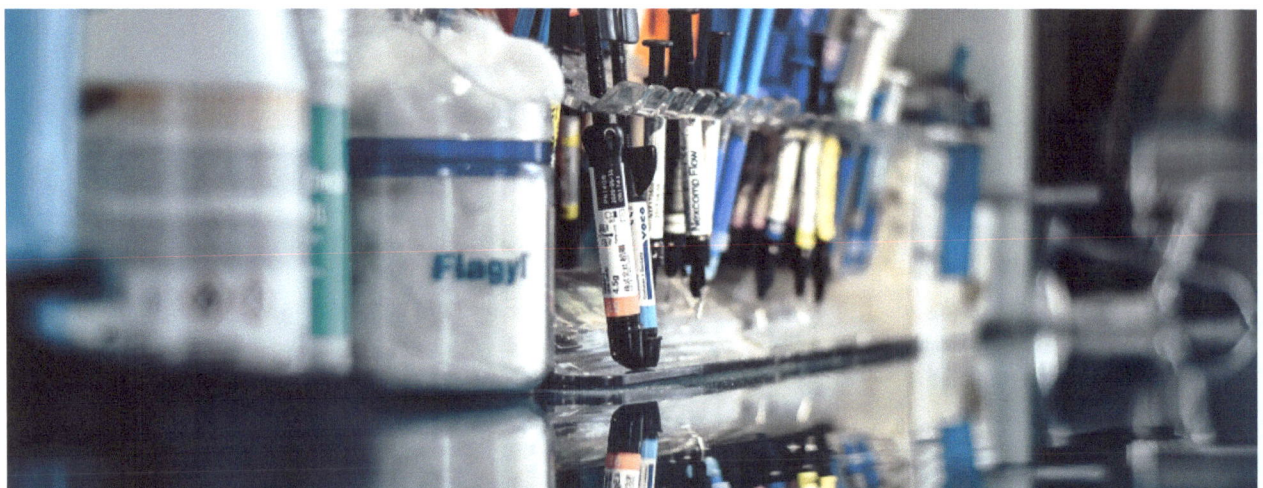

GDT does not consistently result in either increased or decreased amounts of fluid administered. One study showed that the GDT group received more volume. However, in a cohort of septic patients, GDT patients received significantly more fluid during the first six hours than those assigned to standard therapy; but in the overall period from baseline to 72 hours after the start of treatment, there was no significant difference between the two groups in the total amount of fluid administered. Early GDT provided significant outcome benefits: of the patients who survived to hospital discharge, those assigned to standard therapy had significantly longer hospital stays than those with early GDT

Slinger describes one rational approach to fluid administration. The thorax is not assumed to be a third space. Total positive fluid balance in the first 24 hours postoperatively should notexceed20ml/kg or approximately 3L of crystalloid. Unless the patient is at high risk of developing renal insufficiency, urine output of greater than 0.5mL/kg/hr. is probably unnecessary. In the case of reduced tissue perfusion, as in the case of epidural-induced sympathectomy, it is preferable to invasively monitor and use GDT. The use of inotropes may be preferable to aggressive fluid overload.

One limitation of GDT, however, involves the extrapolation of studies correlating cardiac output measurements via PACs with those obtained via dynamic indices during abdominal surgery to thoracotomy patients who are positioned laterally and subjected to varying intrathoracic conditions, such as exposure to atmospheric pressure and OLV.
The value of dynamic preload indicators in the thoracic population has not been systematically examined. Possible problems with extending the use of this device to thoracic surgery patients include lung compliance and intrathoracic pressure variations during positioning changes or insufflation for RATS, laparoscopy and changing intraabdominal pressure, the open chest, pressure changes with VATS, and differing ventilatory settings (TV, PEEP, OLV, DLV).

One study has shown that GDT is at least not deleterious or does not result in pulmonary fluid overload when used for thoracic surgery requiring lateral thoracotomy and OLV.

While changing from the supine to the reverse Trendelenburg or prone positions significantly alters SV and thus SVV,30° left or right recumbent and supine positions do not appear to affect SV or SVV measurements. Kobayashi concludes that SVV, as displayed on the Vigileo monitor, is considered an accurate predictor of intravascular hypovolemia and is a useful indicator for assessing the appropriateness and timing of applying fluid for improving circulatory stability, but only during the perioperative period after esophagectomy.

De Waal (2002) demonstrated that while PiCCO-derived dynamic preload indicators were able to predict fluid responsiveness under closed-chest conditions, both static and dynamic preload indicators failed to predict fluid responsiveness in open-chest conditions.

Stroke volume variation(SVV)and pulse pressure variation (PPV) seem to be critically dependent on the undisturbed transmission of these pressure changes to cardiovascular structures within the closed thorax. For example, sternotomy alone decreases SVV.

Additionally, one study found that SVV could predict fluid responsiveness in patients undergoing OLV with acceptable levels of sensitivity and specificity only when tidal volumes were at least 8mL/kg.

They state that dynamic indices of preload are based on the concept that positive pressure ventilation induces variations in SV. By definition, this concept requires that the preload is significantly affected by cyclic changes in intrathoracic and transpulmonary pressures, and these changes may be too small when patients undergoing OLV are ventilated with low tidal volumes (i.e., 6mL/kg).In short, the ability of SVV to predict volume responsiveness in thoracotomy patients iscurrently unknown.

Finally, the optimal type of fluid is debatable. Some animal models have demonstrated greater interstitial edema with crystalloid administration and better-preserved effective capillary cross-sectional area in the colloid group. Other studies conclude that when given in similar volumes, colloids are more beneficial for anastomotic healing than crystalloids [24, 42].

Improved microcirculatory blood flow and tissue oxygen tension were observed after abdominal surgery in one animal model [60, 61]. However, no difference in anastomotic healing was found in another animal model of colloid use.

To date, no consensus has been reached as to the superiority of crystalloids versus colloids. Pulmonary edema due to excessive crystalloids may clear faster than that caused by colloids.

In summary, intelligent fluid administration is vital to maintaining tissue perfusion and minimizing edema in the perioperative period. New methods of GDT based on SVV may offer useful tools to guide clinicians during thoracic surgery cases. However, the applicability of this technology to the thoracic population has not been fully investigated.

Most likely, avoiding fluid overload by tailoring GDT in an educated manner to the patient's specific deficit and type of fluid loss yields optimal results.

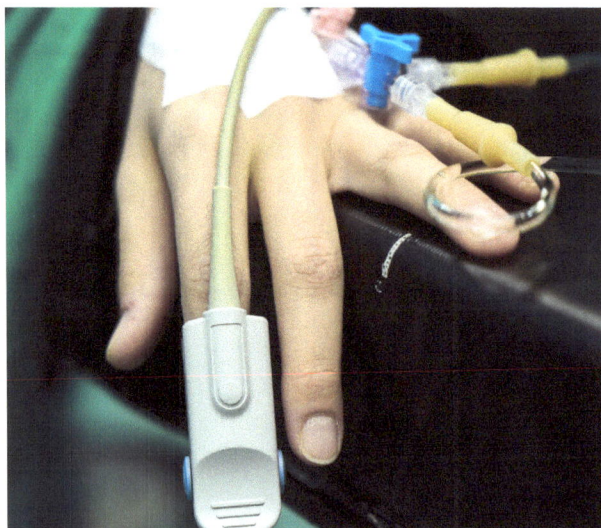

3.3. Special intraoperative monitoring

Since thoracic surgery involves hemodynamic shifts with a goal of tight, goal-directed fluid therapy, knowledge of cardiac output (CO) and fluid responsiveness is important in the perioperative period. The historical gold standard for evaluation of left ventricular end-diastolic pressure (LVEDP), thermodilution (TD) uses a pulmonary artery catheter (PAC) to generate a measured time/temperature curve, from which CO can be calculated. These measurements are averaged over 2-9 minutes, so monitoring is not continuous.

Recent studies show that fluid management based on TD may not improve patient outcomes and may, in fact, increase morbidity and mortality.

PAC use itself may be complicated by arrhythmia, infection, pulmonary artery rupture, and damage to right heart structures. PAC use may be unreliable due to the low-pressure environment of the pulmonary vascular tree and the interference by hydrostatic pressure. With pre-existent pulmonary hypertension, PAC use may become more reliable but conversely have more chance of a complication.

The standard deviation (SD) for TD is about 1 L/minute or about 20% of the average CO . Clearly, reliable and less-invasive methods of measuring CO are needed. Current options include lithium dilution, esophageal Doppler monitoring (EDM), pulse contour cardiac output systems, partialCO2 rebreathing, and thoracic electrical bioimpedance.

Two methods of generating continuous CO measurements require a central venous catheter (CVC), which is arguably invasive, though less so than pulmonary artery catheterization.PiCCO(PULSION Medical Systems AG, Munich, Germany) generates CO via thermodilution from a CVC to a femoral or axillary arterial line. Using the Stewart-Hamilton principle, cold-saline thermodilution is used to provide calibration of the continuous CO analysis.

Similarly, PulseCO (LiDCO Ltd, London, England) uses the Stewart-Hamilton equations as applied to lithium chloride (0.15 - 0.3 mmol for an average adult) dilution from a CVC or peripheral vein to an arterial line.

The arterial lithium concentration-time curve can be subject to error in the presence of certain muscle relaxants. Recalibration is recommended after changes in patient position, therapy, or condition. Clinical studies have demonstrated that over a wide range of cardiac outputs the LiDCOmethod is at least as accurate as thermodilution.

Esophageal doppler monitoring uses a continuous wave sensor on the end of a probe which measures the velocity of blood flow within the descending thoracic aorta. Nomogram estimated aortic cross-sectional area based on the patient's weight, height, and age enables calculation of left ventricular (LV) stroke volume (SV) from the area of the velocity-time waveform.

The total time that blood is traveling in a forward direction within the area is the systolic flow time, which is corrected for heart rate to give the corrected flow time, which is a good index of systemic vascular resistance and is sensitive to changes in LV preload.

There is a positive correlation between measures of cardiac output made simultaneously with the esophageal doppler and a thermodilution PAC.

Limitations of this monitor include assumptions of the diameter of the aorta based on the weight and height of the patient, a learning curve requiring about 12 probe placements, the need for patient sedation, and the inability to be used during esophagectomies.

This method has good validation; however, it only measures aortic blood flow and not true CO, and this may be potentially influenced by disproportionate changes in blood flow between the upper and lower body, although this is only important at the extremes of CO.

Pulse pressure(PP) methods measure the pressure in an artery over time to derive a waveform and use this information to calculate cardiac performance. However, any measure from an artery includes the changes in pressure associated with changes in vascular characteristics such as compliance and impedance. Physiologic or therapeutic changes in vessel diameter seen in the arterial waveform are assumed to reflect changes in CO. The ambiguity of the combined results of CO and vascular tone limits the application of PP methods. The values obtained bytheLiDCOplus can be calibrated daily based on CO values generated by the LiDCO using the CVC waveform. It can also be used independently, as with the FloTrac/Vigileo (EdwardsLifesciences LLC, U.S.A.), which is an uncalibrated pulse contour analysis-based hemodynamic monitor that estimates CO utilizing a standard arterial catheter. The device consists of a pressure transducer which derives a left-sided COfroma sample of arterial pulsations using an algorithm that calculates the product of the standard deviation of the arterial pressure wave (AP) (over 20 seconds) and a vascular tone factor (Khi) to generate stroke volume. Khi is derived from computer analysis of the morphologic change of the arterial pressure waveforms on a bit-by-bit basis based on the principle that changes in compliance or resistance affect the shape of the arterial pressure waveform. The equation in simplified form is as follows:$SV = std(AP) * Khi$ or $BP \times k(constant)$. CO is then derived utilizing the equation $CO = HR * SV$. Only perfused beats that generate an arterial waveform should be counted for HR. While these monitors do not require intracardiac catheterization with a pulmonary artery catheter, they do require an arterial line. The benefit of this technology includes the short time required for set up and data acquisition.

Disadvantages include its inability to provide right-sided heart pressures or mixed venous oxygen saturation. In addition, arterial monitoring systems are unable to predict changes in vascular tone and can therefore only estimate changes in vascular compliance.

Some consider the measurement of pressure in the artery to calculate flow in the heart physiologically over-simplified and of questionable accuracy and benefit [64, 69]. The sensor is only indicated for adult use and has not been validated in patients with ventricular assist devices or intra-aortic balloon pumps.

Absolute values during aortic regurgitation may be affected although trending may be appropriate. This monitor is dependent upon a high-fidelity pressure tracing, which is compromised by spontaneous ventilation, atrial fibrillation or ectopy, severe peripheral constriction with vasopressor use, hypothermia, or dynamic autonomic states such as sepsis. In those instances, femoral artery cannulation or insertion of a PAC may be considered.

Finally, in a study comparing these devices, although the PAC, FloTrac, LiDCO, and PiCCOdisplay similar mean CO values, they trended differently in response to therapy and showed different inter-device agreements. In the clinically relevant low CO range (< 5 L/min), agreement improved slightly. Thus, utility and validation studies using only one CO device may potentially not be extrapolated to equivalency of using another similar device

The Fick principle allows multiple substitutions for O2 consumption, including CO2 clearance. Based on the ratio of the change in end-tidal CO2 (etCO2) and CO2 elimination, the Noninvasive Cardiac Output (NICO) device (Novametrix Medical Systems, Inc., Wallingford, CT, USA) calculates CO using a disposable rebreathing loop which allows intermittent partial rebreathing in 3-minute cycles.

This system contains a CO2 sensor which uses infrared light absorption, a disposable airflow sensor or differential pressure pneumotachometer, a specific disposable rebreathing loop, and a pulse oximeter.

The production of CO2 (VCO2, mL/min) is calculated from minute ventilation and its instantaneous CO2 content, where the CaCO2 (mL/100 mL of blood) is estimated from etCO2 (mmHg).

The rebreathing cycle induces an increase in etCO2 and mimics a drop in CO2 production. CO2 production is calculated as the product of CO2 concentration and airflow during a breathing cycle, and the arterial content of CO2 (CaCO2)isderivedfromtheetCO2 and the CO2 dissociation curve.

The obtained differences of these values are then used to calculate CO,
such that
CO=ΔVCO2/(S x Δet CO2),
where S is the slope of the CO2 dissociation curve. The NICO system provides rapid, reliable CO values for mechanically ventilated patients with minor lung abnormalities and stable ventilatory settings.

The NICO system is also limited. For example, intrapulmonary shunt can affect the estimation of CO. Also, in patients undergoing thoracic surgery with OLV, the device underestimated CO compared with thermodilution CO at all measurement times.

With worsening pulmonary injury or hemodynamic compromise contributing to increasing shunt and dead space, assumptions made for calculating CO are less likely to approximate actual values. This technique reliably measures CO in patients affected by diseases causing low levels of pulmonary shunt, but underestimates it in patients with shunt higher than 35%.

In summary, compared to TD methods, the partial CO2 rebreathing technique is non-invasive, can easily be automated, and can provide real-time and continuous cardiac output monitoring. Largeoutcome studies demonstrating the use of this device are still lacking.

Impedance cardiography (ICG) or thoracic electrical bioimpedance (TEB) uses changes in thoracic impedance over the cardiac cycle to generate CO. A constant magnitude, high frequency, low amplitude current is applied longitudinally across a segment of the thorax. Using Ohm's Law, the voltage difference within the current field is proportional to the electrical impedance (Z).

Contraction of the heart produces a cyclical change in transthoracic impedance of about 0.5%. Upon ventricular ejection, a time-dependent cardiac-synchronous pulsatile impedance change is observed, $\Delta Z(t)$, which constitutes the time-variable total transthoracic impedance $Z(t)$, when electrically parallel to baseline impedance ($Z0$).

Lower impedance indicates greater intrathoracic fluid volume and blood flow. TEB has waveform characteristics representing points in the cardiac cycle.

The first derivative (dz/dt) of the waveform is used to identify the maximum upslope point, which is used to calculate the Velocity Index (VI). The VI is indicative of aortic blood velocity, such that impaired contractility is reflected by a decreased VI. By synchronizing fluid volume changes with the cardiac cycle, the change in

impedance can be used to calculate SV, CO, and systemic vascular resistance. TEB equipment consists of both noninvasive and invasive devices, of which the former has gained more acceptance.

Examples include the Bio-Z Dx (Sonosite Inc®, Bothell, WA) and theniccomo® (medis GmbH, Ilmenau, Germany). Some studies comparing TEB-derived CO to TD have found significant correlation between the methods, but inaccuracies were observed with severe tachycardia, low CO, or frequent arrhythmias [75].

Questions with respect to the reliability and validity of this technique have led some to advocate its use only in research settings [76]. The clinical use of TEBhas yet to be established.

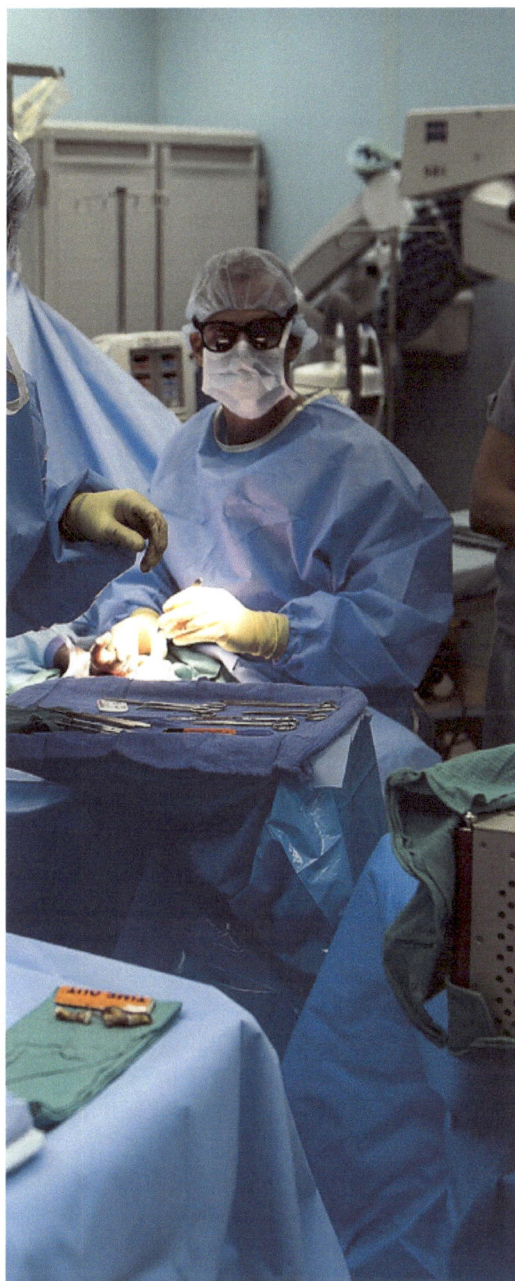

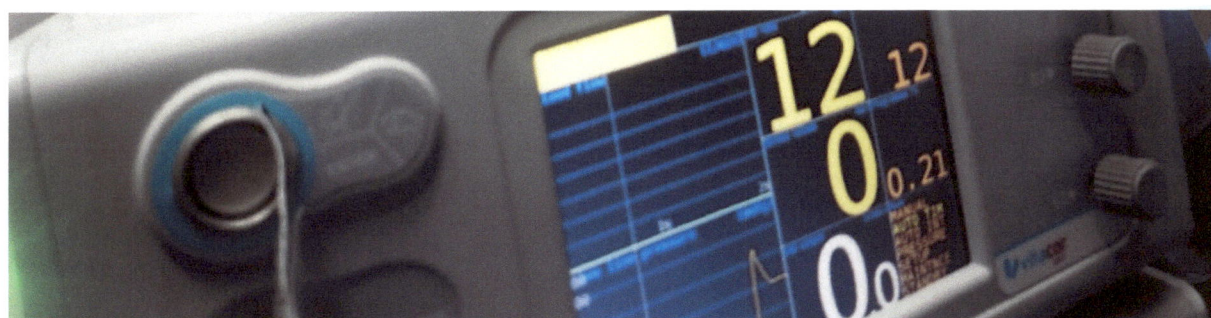

Transesophageal echocardiography (TEE) is a method of ultrasound-based cardiac imaging which allows real-time visualization of anatomic structure and function. In the specific setting of thoracic surgery, TEE can be used to monitor ventricular function, valvular function, and wall motion changes reflective of ischemia during positioning changes, volume shifts, OLV, or surgical resection. Intrathoracic tumors may be visible in some exams, and compression or infiltration of structures such as the pulmonary artery or innominate vein may be visualized. Tumor invasion of the heart may be appreciated, as can other anatomic abnormalities resulting from the underlying disease process or iatrogenic causes.

Intraoperative hemodynamic instability of unknown cause and the need for evaluation of affected cardiac and pulmonary structures will likely satisfy the Appropriate Use Criteria for Echocardiography [77].

Commoncontraindications to TEE use include some features present in the thoracic surgery population such as known esophageal strictures, perforation, lacerations or large diverticula. Relative contraindications also obviate TEE use in esophagectomies: dysphagia or odynophagia, recentupperGI bleeding, extensive radiation to the chest and mediastinum, and esophageal varices.

In terms of global cardiac function, the transgastric short-axis and right ventricular ejection fraction. Calculation of CO is also possible with two-dimensional(2D)Doppler measurements, such that CO = Aortic valve area (AVA) x heart rate (HR) x velocity time integral (TVI).AVA may be measured by planimetry of the AV via the mid esophageal AV short axis view, with the imaging plane at approximately 30°.

Another common method of calculating AVA is with the continuity equation, which states that the flow in one area must equal the flow in a second area if there are no shunts between the two areas. In practical terms, the flow from the left ventricular outflow tract (LVOT) is compared to the flow at the level of the aortic valve:

Aortic Valve Area (cm2)= LVOT diametert x 0.78540 x1LVOT TV 1
Where the CSA LVOT(cm2) = 0.785 x LVOTDiameter2
TVI is an integral of instantaneous blood flow velocities during one cardiac cycle. To measure the LVOT TVI, the pulsed-Doppler sample volume is positioned just proximal to the aortic valve so that the location of the velocity recording matches the LVOT diameter measurement.

When the sample volume is optimally positioned, the recording shows a smooth velocity curve with a well-defined peak and narrow band of velocities throughout systole. The TVI is measured by tracing the dense modal velocity throughout systole. The same is done for the AV TVI.

TEE assessment of cardiac and intrathoracic structures and functions is a clinically established method that plays a critical role in the diagnosis and management of perioperative hemodynamic instability in many institutions [78].

However, its main disadvantage is that its use requires extensive training and a skilled operator. Some measurements may be challenging to acquire and subject to methodical error or inability to obtain images adequately parallel to the ultrasound plane. Hemodynamic measurements obtained with TEE compared to TD with a PAC have resulted in agreements ranging from good [79] to possessing"accuracy limitations" [80].

A significant source of this inconsistency may result from interoperator variability.

Further, in the instance of thoracic cases, proper contact with the stomach and esophagus in the lateral position can hinder the acquisition of adequate images.
Other inconveniences include the expense of the equipment and the fact that an image cannot be easily fixed in order to provide continuous cardiac output readings without the presence of an expert user.

In summary, the physiologic and hemodynamic challenges inherent to thoracic surgery may require not only monitoring via an arterial wave pressure measurement but possibly other modalities as well. PAC, lithium dilution, EDM, pulse contour cardiac output systems, partial CO_2 rebreathing, TEB, and TEE constitute such alternatives. While validation of these methods may be forthcoming,reasonable application of these modalities may improve perioperative management and overall patient outcomes.

3.4. Special operative scenarios and anesthetic considerations

3.4.1. VATSversus open thoracotomy

The decision as to whether a particular surgery can be performed using a video-assisted thoracoscopic or an open thoracotomy approach is a decision usually made by the surgeon. In 2007, at the International Society of Minimally Invasive Cardiothoracic Surgery conference, evidence revealed that VATS can be recommended to reduce overall postoperative complications, can reduce pain and overall functionality over the short term, improve delivery of adjuvant chemotherapy delivery, and can be recommended for lobectomy in clinical stage I and II non-small cell lung cancer patients. The recommendations were based on data derived from single and multiple randomized studies, but with conflicting evidence and/or divergence of opinion about the usefulness or efficacy of the procedure [81]. No general consensus using multiple randomized clinical trials has been done as to the preference of surgical technique. The bottom line is that with the learning curve for the VATS procedure, individual surgeons choose their own preferred method of surgical intervention. The role of an anesthesiologist is to be prepared for any lung surgery, both of which usually encompass one-lung ventilation, either through a double-lumen tube or a bronchial blocker as a general anesthetic. A minorVATSprocedure such as pleural biopsy or thoracentesis can actually be done with local anesthesia +/- intravenous sedation [82].

These procedures are rare in the operating room, however, and most VATS procedures are in actuality done under general anesthesia. An endobronchial ultrasound is done at our institute in the pulmonary lab as a general anesthetic with a laryngeal mask airway.

Although a single-lumen endotracheal tube can be used under general anesthesia for open thoracotomy, the operative lung field would also undergo positive pressure ventilation, making it technically more difficult for the surgeon. In small infants, a balloon-tipped bronchial blocker can be placed to isolate the lungmer[83] or placing ETT into the mainstem of the nonoperative lung are also other options if a double lumen tube is too large to be placed.

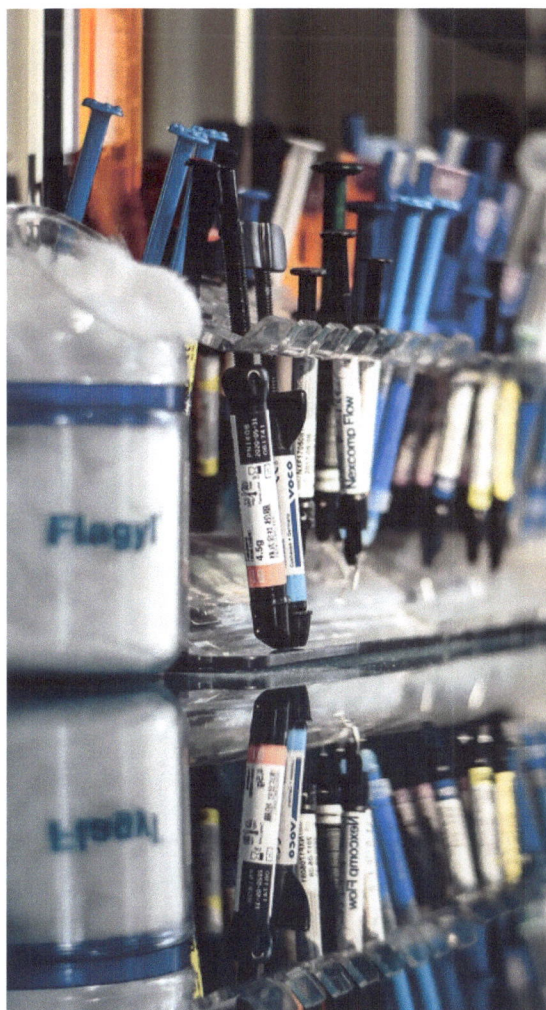

It is estimated that double lung tube placement has resulted in iatrogenic injuryin0.5-2per 1000 cases of DLT placement[84], so care must be made to decrease these complications. One advantage of a double lumen tube above a bronchial blocker is the ability to suction out the operable lung if and when necessary and increased intraoperative stability with the tube itself.

The bronchial blocker is often difficult to obtain lung isolation in the right lung due to the takeoff of the right upper lobe being so close to the carina, but this technique is necessary to understand in case a double lumen is unable to be placed (in patients with abnormal anatomy) [85], or if a patient is already intubated with a single lumen tube with a difficult airway and need slung isolation.

There have been a number of cases where both are used successfully, however. The key is having the lung isolated, and understanding physiology to understand how to utilize hypoxic pulmonary vasoconstriction to each patient's advantage.

In a thoracoscopic procedure, the surgeon does not have the ability to push the operative lung out of his/her way like an open thoracotomy.

Thus, the importance of the lung being deflated is made apparent. Sometimes, a suction catheter can be placed in the operable lung to facilitate deflation of the lung. It is important to know if the surgeon is to insufflate with carbon dioxide so that complications of insufflation can also be recognized. A VATS procedure is, although for the patient sometimes easier to manage postoperatively, for the surgeon and anesthesiologist comes with various difficulties.

One of these difficulties has to do with not having enough access or visualization in cases where the pulmonary artery or another major vessel is inadvertently traumatized and the patient is bleeding. Therefore, it is always important to have blood available for a possible blood transfusion in both open thoracotomies and VATSprocedures.

An arterial line is necessary to keep a close eye on thermodynamics during both types of procedures. The positioning for both usually entails a lateral decubitus position, and pressure points must be checked. The postoperative pain level for patients with a thoracoscopic procedure is usually less than the open thoracotomy patient though this has been questioned. Chronic pain rates may be similar with VATS and open thoracotomies. A status post VATS procedure patient can achieve pain control with IV medications, while an epidural is usually recommended for thoracotomy patients. These methods of pain control will be discussed in a later chapter.

3.4.2. Airway disruptive surgeries

Airway disruptive surgeries require special communication between the surgeon and anesthesiologist as to what is going to be required intraoperatively. With surgical and an esthetic advances, now more than half the trachea can be safely excised in selected cases[86]. A tracheal resection is something done rarely, requiring the anesthesiologist and surgeon to share the airway. The type of anesthetic utilized depends on the skill of the anesthesiologist, and the experience within each independent institution, as to the Bestway to carry out this surgical procedure.

There have been many case reports depicting many different methods of maintaining oxygenation and ventilation for a patient while still undergoing thoracic procedure that compromises the trachea or bronchus.
The main anesthetic concern is always adequate ventilation and oxygenation when the airway is essentially open. It is also important to both the anesthesiologist and surgeon to protect the integrity of the new tracheal anastomosis postoperatively. Steroids are often given to help decrease airway edema. A high FiO2 is necessary to help maintain oxygenation during periods of ventilatory pauses, but a close eye should be kept on electrocautery use. If indeed it is being used, then the lowest FiO2 that the patient can tolerate should be kept to help prevent airway fire. An arterial line is a good monitor to check for innominate compression (such as in a medianstinoscopy) during surgical dissection

A technique where a laryngeal mask airway is utilized with high-frequency jet ventilation for a patient with tracheal stenosis has also been reported. In this otherwise healthy patient with tracheal stenosis from prolonged intubation, an LMA was placed and the patient was put on positive pressure ventilation.

A sterile 6-mm flexible tube was placed in the distal trachea and the patient adequately oxygenated/ventilated while the dissection and lesion was resected. Once the tracheal anastomosis started, a jet ventilator was placed in the distal trachea and the patient jet-ventilated for tracheal anastomosis.

Once completed, the patient was once again placed on positive pressure ventilation through the LMA while the patient was awakened, found adequately spontaneously ventilating, and extubated successfully[87].

There are disadvantages to using high-frequency jet ventilation such as during exhalation there may be air trapping from the stenotic lesion, the catheter could become occluded by blood and displaced, and there might be distal aspiration of debris or blood[88].

More routinely, an endotracheal tube can be placed above the area of stenosis. Once surgical exposure is done, a separate tube can be placed distal to the stricture and the patient placed on the ventilator with sterility across the field. Once the trachea is resected, the primary endotracheal tube can be passed distal to the lesion and the anastomosis completed.

Another case has been reported in a patient with critical trachea stenosis. The patient underwent femoral-femoral extracorporeal bypass prior to induction. An endotracheal tube was placed after induction, and the patient was maintained on the endotracheal tube and positive pressure ventilation as he/she was weaned from the cardiopulmonary bypass machine.

A prospective study has been done in patients with upper tracheal stenosis that were managed with a cervical epidural anesthesia, local anesthesia and conscious sedation while maintaining spontaneous ventilation throughout the resection[90].

Although only twenty consecutive patients were enrolled, the outcome had a high level of patient satisfaction and immediate feedback from the patient throughout the procedure. This bypasses the need for jet ventilation or positive pressure ventilation, and enables communication with the patient throughout the surgical procedure.

Post resection, usually the patient is extubated with their neck in a flexed position to put less tension on the anastomosis.

Not infrequently the patients chin is sutured to the manubrium sterni with a heavy stitch to maintain the flexion. A smooth extubation with minimal coughing/bucking is preferred for the same reason. Extubation is important post operatively to reduce the positive pressure on the suture line as well. Pain control is often not an issue, a tracheal resection is not a very painful procedure, and intravenous narcotics and local anesthesia should be adequate for control.

3.4.3. Endotracheal tube exchange (Double to single lumen tube exchange)

These days, double lumen tubes are routinely used for surgeries requiring lung isolation. If extubation is unable to be accomplished at the conclusion of the surgery, the decision must be made to either keep the double lumen in place, or exchange it for a single lumen tube. Lessthan1% of patients, however, require mechanical ventilation after surgery[91].

Exchanging the double lumen tube avoids the potential obstruction of the airway that can occur when secretions/blood get lodged in the bronchial tube. Also, the nursing staff that is to be taking care of the patient postoperatively might not understand how to troubleshoot a double lumen endobronchial tube, so misuse of the tube may occur including airway rupture.

Exchanging a double-lumen endobronchial tube to a single-lumen endotracheal tube has many considerations and should be approached with some trepidation.

An airway that was initially easy to place the double lumen in might not be easy after the surgery with volume shifts and edema. If it is thought the airway might be lost in the exchange, leaving the double lumen in overnight with the head of the bed elevated to help alleviate edema might be the safest option.

It has been shown that the flow resistances of modern double lumen tubes are actually much lower than previously supposed, so the need to change them is not as important during spontaneous ventilation and weaning from the ventilator as previously thought[92].

The effective diameter of each lumen of an adult double lumen endobronchial tube is comparable to a 6.0-7.0 mm outside diameter ETT [93], so adequate oxygenation/ventilation is manageable without exchanging the tube. If an exchange is necessary, there are a few options described.

The first option is using a tube exchanger to facilitate the exchange of the double lumen tube to a single lumen.

First, adequate anesthesia and suctioning down both lumens of the double lumen should be done. FiO2 should be 1.0. A tube exchanger is placed after being lubricated through the tracheal lumen, both cuffs are deflated, and the double lumen is removed over the stylet.

A single lumen is then placed, sometimes while performing a direct laryngoscopy to facilitate the exchange. There are other scenarios described using the Eschmann stylet as a tube exchanger in various alternative ways [94].

The easiest and quickest method to exchanging the tube is just by performing a direct laryngoscopy after the patient is adequately anesthetized. If visualization of the cords is easy while the double lumen is still in place, it can be withdrawn and a single lumen placed under direct visualization.

Whichever technique is chosen, the safety of the patient comes first. If it is unsafe to change the tube out, an alternative is to just pull out the double lumen so the bronchial cuff is in the trachea, thus operating as a single lumen tube. Understanding that the airway anatomy and ease of visualization might not be the same as it was preoperatively is very important. Certainly it will not improve.

3.4.4. Post-operative need for bronchoscopy prior to emergence

Certain surgical scenarios may require fiber optic bronchoscopic examination after completion of the surgical procedure, but prior to patient emergence (if extubation is planned).

These scenarios include the examination of the integrity of anastomotic sites, the examination of anatomic structures (e.g.. the vocal cords) to ensure proper postoperative function, and the clearing of debris (tissue, secretions, and blood) from the proximal and distal airways.

During fiberoptic bronchoscopic examination, the anesthesiologist must meticulously plan airway control techniques to ensure an optimal environment for bronchoscopy as well as adequate patient oxygenation and ventilation.

When a single-lumen endotracheal tube (SLT) is already in use, the procedure is usually straightforward. If a bronchial blocker is used in combination with an SLT for lung isolation, one simply removes the blocker from the SLT to facilitate fiber-optic bronchoscopy (bronchoscopy could also be performed with the blocker in place, if needed).

However, one must keep in mind that the internal diameter of the indwelling SLT must be large enough to accommodate an appropriately sized bronchoscope, especially if adequate suction (provided by larger bronchoscopes) is required to clear debris.

When a double-lumen endotracheal tube (DLT) is used for lung isolation, the procedure is more complicated. Fiberoptic bronchoscopy with a DLT in place is difficult because of the specialized tube's design and required positioning. First, the internal diameters of the dual lumens of the DLT are small. This limits the size of bronchoscopes that maybe used(3.6-4.9mmouterdiameter)—smaller bronchoscopes do not provide the view or possess the suctioning capabilities of larger bronchoscopes.

Second, DLTs are considerably longer and more invasive than conventional SLTs. DLTs are positioned (post intubation) so that the distal opening of the tracheal lumen closely abuts the primary carina with the distal bronchial end placed in the appropriate mainstem bronchi (for which the DLT was designed).

Therefore, a properly placed DLT restricts direct bronchoscopic examination of a majority of the trachea and mainstem bronchi. Comprehensive bronchoscopic examination in this scenario requires removal of the DLT and subsequent replacement with an SLT or supraglottic airway device(e.g. Laryngeal Mask Airway TM - LMA North America, San Diego, CA, U.S.A.) in an anesthetized patient.

Supraglotticairwaydevicesdonotrequireendotrach ealintubationandarepreferredover reintubation with an SLT because they reduce the possibility of trauma to fresh surgical anastomosis sites within the airways, improve the visualization of proximal airway structures – vocal cords, proximal trachea – that would be otherwise obstructed by SLTs, accommodate larger bronchoscopes for improved visualization and suctioning, and are less complicated to place than SLTs and do not require neuromuscular blockade for easy placement.

In patients with non-difficult airways, supraglottic airway devices may be immediately placed after deep extubation (in a blind fashion). In patients with difficult airways, supraglottic airway devices may be pre-positioned posterior to the DLT prior to extubation.

This allows for fiber-optic visual confirmation of the device's proper positioning (by continuous visualization of the glottic opening) prior to, during, and after extubation. Once the positioning of the supraglottic airway device and adequate ventilation are confirmed, fiberoptic examination of the airways may proceed. Upon completion of the bronchoscopic exam, the patient may be emerged from anesthesia with the device in place without the need for reintubation.

3.4.5. Pulmonary procedures in out-of-O.R. settings

A trend is growing toward performing pulmonary procedures in specialized non-O.R. pulmonary procedure suites, rather than the traditional operating room. These procedures may be performed for diagnostic or therapeutic purposes and include flexible/rigid bronchoscopy, pleuroscopy, tracheo-bronchial stent placement or dilation, and endobronchial ultrasound-guided lymph node sampling [95]. In these settings, special anesthetic considerations must be made regarding choice of agents, airway devices, and ventilatory modes.

a.   Agents

A total intravenous anesthetic (TIVA) approach is the most practical mode of anesthetic delivery in these settings. A TIVA-based approach avoids volatile anesthetic agents that could be lost from airways in procedures that involve a breach of the airway (and/or the airway device).

Loss of agent through a breach could result in inadequate anesthetic levels, exposure of personnel to volatile agents, combustion and airway fire (N2O), or production of toxic products after pyrolysis. Furthermore, special ventilatory modes (such as jet-ventilation)necessary for certain pulmonary procedures preclude the use of volatile anesthetics.

Two anesthetic challenges during pulmonary procedures are providing adequate anesthesia during alternating periods of high and low stimulation (in which anesthetic requirements also fluctuate rapidly), and rapid recovery post-procedure [96]. The intravenous agents propofol, remifentanil, and lidocaine have specific advantages in these situations, primarily as a result of their pharmacokinetic/pharmacodynamic profiles.

The standard sedative-hypnotic for TIVA administration is propofol, and, in fact, propofol is the only sedative-hypnotic that is used on a standard basis for continuous infusion. Only propofol has the combination of quick onset, short half-life, rapid redistribution, amnesia, effective airway reflex depression, wide anesthetic depth range, and antiemetic properties.

It does not, however, provide analgesia; therefore, narcotics are usually added to a TIVA regimen. Narcotics provide analgesia, reduce the propofol dosage needed, and also suppress the cough reflex.

Remifentanil is an ultra-short acting narcotic (context-sensitive half-life: 3-5 minutes) that is metabolized by nonspecific tissue and plasma esterases; therefore, it is ideal intraoperatively to manage moments of high stimulation while avoiding over-accumulation of narcotic when stimulation subsides [97].

In patients for whom post-procedure pain control or cough suppression is needed, a longer-acting narcotic may be co-administered with remifentanil. Lastly, intravenous lidocaine is a useful adjunct to propofol and remifentanil in TIVA. Lidocaine is an amide-type local anesthetic that reduces the need for both propofol and narcotics; it also suppresses airway reflexes and is an effective post-procedure anti-tussive.

b.   Airway devices

Airway management for pulmonary procedures must address the need for adequate patient oxygenation/ventilation, permit complete examination of areas of interest of the airway, and accommodate the necessary diagnostic and/or interventional instruments needed for the procedure. In most cases, supraglottic airways (e.g., Laryngeal Mask Airway TM) meet these requirements and are the airway devices of choice.

They are easy to place without the need for specialized equipment, are an integral part of the standard difficult airway algorithm, may be used in spontaneously or mechanically ventilated patients, and provide limited airway protection from regurgitation.

Furthermore, supraglottic airways may be easily used as a bridge in a case where definitive airway control will be managed via rigid bronchoscopy/jet-ventilation. In such a case, the supraglottic airway is placed as a temporary airway conduit during induction, is removed once the rigid bronchoscopy begins, and is replaced at the end of the procedure to serve as the airway conduit until emergence from anesthesia.

c. Ventilatory modes

Patient ventilation/oxygenation during pulmonary procedures may be spontaneous or mechanical, depending on the requirements of the procedure. Adequacy of oxygenation and ventilation is measured by pulse oximetry and end-tidal CO_2 measurement.

It is important to note that while end-tidal CO_2 detection is vital in confirming adequate ventilation, it is often inconsistent due to airway breach and suctioning inherent during pulmonary procedures. Of the various mechanical ventilation modes, jet-ventilation deserves particular attention. Jet-ventilation is typically associated with rigid bronchoscopy. In this situation, total airway control will be in the hands of the interventionalist/surgeon, with the anesthesiologist controlling the jet-ventilator.

Control of jet ventilation may be by automated jet delivery systems or manually by the anesthesiologist. Automated systems have several benefits over manual delivery, including greater control of delivered FiO_2 and respiratory frequency, duration, and flow. Additionally, automation gives anesthesia personnel greater freedom to attend to other aspects of the anesthetic care.

3.4.6. Post anesthesia recovery considerations for patients undergoing thoracic procedures

The immediate post-operative care of the thoracic surgical patient is focused on ensuring conditions that optimize oxygenation/ventilation and recognizing possible post-operative complications inherent to thoracic surgery.

a.   Extubation

If feasible, immediate post-operative extubation is favored to avoid unnecessary hemodynamic stress, the disruption of fresh surgical sites from continued intubation, positive-pressure ventilation, and/or coughing, and the development of ventilator-associated pneumonia [99].

However, the tentative respiratory condition of the typical thoracic surgery patient warrants careful consideration when making the decision to extubate (see preoperative anesthetic evaluation above).

The physician must not only optimize routine respiratory criteria for extubation – pH $\geq$ 7.30, $FiO_2 \leq$ 0.4-0.5, $PaO_2/FiO_2 >$ 150-200, PEEP $\leq$ 5-8 cmH2O, RR $\leq$ 30 bpm, $SpO_2 \geq$ 90%, $PaO_2 \geq$ 60, $PaCO_2 \leq$ 50, Vt > 5 ml/kg, VC >15 ml/kg, NIF > -20 cm H2O – but must also recognize the variable nature of emergence from anesthesia and consider the state of other important clinical variables [100].

These variables include the ability to follow commands, the return of airway protective reflexes, adequate reversal of neuromuscular blockade (with good motor strength), adequate pain control, normothermia, hemodynamic stability, and normal electrolyte values.

Additionally, the rapid shallow breathing index (RSBI - the ratio of respiratory frequency to tidal volume (f/VT)) combines superior sensitivity (97%) and negative predictive value (95%) when predicting weaning success.

Once extubation is achieved, the focus is on optimizing pulmonary physiology; three fundamental measures are essential. First, supplemental oxygen should be administered and adequate ventilation confirmed, because hypoxia and hypercarbia are well known to increase pulmonary vascular resistance [103].

Second, the patient should be positioned supine with the head of the bed elevated (semi-Fowler's position) to lessen the risk of aspiration and decrease the work of breathing. Third, pain control must be evaluated; pain increases sympathetic tone, elevating pulmonary artery pressures and pulmonary vascular resistance, and elicits respiratory splinting that limits ventilation and results in hypercapnia.

In some cases, continued intubation and mechanical ventilation is required postoperatively. Under these circumstances, it is important to achieve the transition from positive pressure to spontaneous ventilation as quickly as possible. In addition, extubation criteria should be assessed frequently so that extubation may be acheived as soon as possible.

b. Post-operative Complications

Operations involving vital thoracic structures place patients at higher risk of life-threatening post-operative complications. An in-depth discussion of these complications can be found in chapters detailing the post-operative course of these patients. This section focuses on select complications that may occur in the immediate post-operative recovery period: injuries in the conducting airways, pneumothorax, and cardiac herniation.

i.   Injuries in the conducting airways

Advanced anesthetic airway management and surgical manipulation predispose the thoracic surgery patient to a variety of post-operative airway complications. Injuries range from erythema/edema (most commonly) to vocal cord injuries and tracheo-bronchial rupture (TBR) (rarely).

Supportive therapy with supplemental humidified oxygen is adequate for mild symptoms of airway edema; however, constant monitoring for worsening respiratory obstruction is paramount. Iatrogenic vocal cord injuries resulting from intubation and/or damage to the recurrent laryngeal nerve may lead to airway compromise and increase risk of aspiration, if the damage is bilateral.

Dyspnea, stridor, and inability to phonate are symptoms commonly associated with bilateral vocal cord injury/paralysis. If respiratory distress is present, the airway should be definitely controlled via intubation or tracheostomy. TBR caused by DLT intubation is extremely rare, with a reported incidence of less than 0.5 % [84]. Hemoptysis and subcutaneous crepitus (in the neck and upper chest area) are the most common presenting symptoms with respiratory distress and/or collapse occurring in advanced cases [104]. If TBR is suspected and surgical intervention planned, general anesthesia should be induced while preferably maintaining spontaneous ventilation to avoid worsening of the injury by barotrauma. Initial airway control with a supraglottic airway is preferred, when possible, to avoid further injury that can occur with endotracheal intubation.

Further, a supraglottic airway allows for complete fiber-optic examination of the trachea, bronchi, and distal airways. Fiber-optic examination of the tracheobronchial tree is important to confirm the diagnosis of TBR and to locate the lesion.

Once the location and extent of the injury is determined, the type and application of airway control may be chosen and surgical repair undertaken. In extreme situations, cardio-pulmonary bypass maybe required to assure oxygenation and ventilation.

ii.   Pneumothorax

Pneumothorax is a potentially grave immediate postoperative complication that may necessitate prompt intervention. The creation of a pneumothorax is inherent in any procedure involving the breach of the thoracic cavity. The severity of pneumothorax is determined by its magnitude and whether it is in communication externally with atmospheric pressure.

A pneumothorax of small volume is usually well tolerated; however, with increased magnitude, it exerts considerable effects to the heart and vasculature in the confined space of the thoracic cavity. These may lead to hemodynamic collapse and respiratory compromise – a tension pneumothorax. Chest drainage tubes are used to decrease the magnitude of a pneumothorax by providing an avenue of escape for trapped air (and/or blood, secretions, etc.) from the thoracic cavity. Specialized "balanced" drainage systems have been developed for certain operations, such as pneumonectomy.

Balanced systems provide a buffer to prevent excessive negative or positive intrathoracic pressures from developing, lowering the chance for both tension pneumothorax and cardiac herniation (see below) [105]. In circumstances where chest tubes are not placed or where the drainage system malfunctions, tension pneumothorax may develop. In this scenario, intrathoracic pressures must be relieved immediately via needle decompression and/or emergent chest tube insertion. One must recognize that contralateral pneumothorax is also a possibility from anesthetic (contralateral central venous catheters, epidural (paramedian) placement, barotrauma) as well as surgical (breach of the contralateral pleura) insult [106]. Care must be taken to avoid clamping chest tubes after thoracotomy to avoid formation of a pneumothorax.

iii.   Cardiac herniation

Cardiac herniation, although rare, is a potentially fatal postoperative complication most commonly associated with disruption of the pericardium – most commonly during the course of or after a pneumonectomy.

The usual presenting symptoms are generalized hypotension and tachycardia; however, right versus left sided cardiac herniation may present with additional distinct signs and symptoms inherent to the physiologic disruption unique to the direction of herniation [107, 108]. Leftward herniation places the heart at risk for myocardial ischemia and arrhythmias, because of the potential constriction of the ventricles by pericardial tissue during the course of the herniation [107, 108].

Rightward herniation predisposes the patient to superior vena cava (SVC) syndrome – head, neck and upper-extremity cyanosis, edema, etc. - secondary to torsion and obstruction of the SVC and inadequate cardiac preload because of impaired venous drainage [107, 108]. After assessing signs and symptoms, cardiac herniation may be confirmed via imaging - chest x-ray and/or echocardiography. Immediate surgical intervention to reduce the herniation and correct the pericardial defect is paramount to prevent further hemodynamic collapse [107, 108].

The gravity of cardiac herniation warrants recovery measures to help minimize its occurrence. Avoid patient positioning with the operative side dependent, to reduce gravitational effects favoring herniation.

As discussed above, early extubation is favored to alleviate the effects of positive pressure ventilation and its tendency to instigate and worsen herniation. Lastly, avoid negative pressure via chest drainage tubes (preferably using balanced chest drainage systems in pneumonectomies) to minimize a vacuum effect that may predispose to herniation.

4. Pain management for the thoracic surgical patient

4.1. Post-thoracotomy pain syndrome

Thoracotomies continue to cause substantial pain because of the degree of surgical injury. Insult to the intercostal nerves, soft tissue damage and inflammation, bone and joint disturbance, and visceral manipulation all contribute to the severity of pain[88]. The estimated incidence of chronic pain following thoracotomy is between 30-40%, with approximately 10%withsevere disabling pain [109, 110]. Pain control is crucial after thoracic surgery not only for immediate pain relief, but also to prevent pulmonary complications.

"Pain that recurs or persists along a thoracotomy scar at least two months following the surgical procedure" [111] is the definition of post-thoracotomy pain syndrome (PTPS). Poor pain management after thoracotomy may contribute to PTPS [112]. The pain is largely described as aching, with tenderness and numbness at or around the surgical incision/scar[113].In contrast to acute pain, which mostly affects respiratory function, PTPS may be responsible for inability to perform daily activities. Although PTPS likely plays a negative role in daily life, its impact is unclear because these subjective phenomena have not been reliably assessed.

Although video assisted thoracic surgery (VATS) was anticipated to reduce pain when compared to traditional posterolateral thoracotomy, its smaller port sites do not necessarily avoid intercostal nerve injury owing to aggressive manipulation of the scopes and instruments. The pain associated with VATS is not significantly different to that of thoracotomy[115] and there are conflicting differences in the incidence of PTPS [113, 114]. It is unclear if patients with preventative analgesia by way of thoracic epidural analgesia have fewer propensities to develop PTPS [114]. Other regional techniques have not yet been studied in this capacity [114]. There is also conflicting evidence of the causality of acute pain on.

There are many modalities of postoperative pain control that will be briefly explained here.

4.2. Systemic analgesics

Opioids have a long-standing history of providing effective pain relief. It is the unwanted side-effects that discourage their use including: nausea, vomiting, respiratory depression, ileus, biliary spasms, urinary retention, sedation, and pruritis. Opioids can be given by many routes– oral, intravenous, intramuscular, transdermal, transmucosal. Intravenous patient controlled analgesia (PCA) allows for increased safety, less opioid use, ability to titrate to individual needs, and some increase in patient satisfaction [116]. Using opioids alone may lead to intolerable side effects, which has led to the concomitant use of other drug classes for their synergistic effects.

Ketamine is an N-methyl-D-aspartate (NMDA) antagonist that has direct spinal effects as well as depresses the thalamus and activates the limbic system. It acts at the phencyclidine binding site and has been used as an induction agent. At lower doses, it provides effective analgesia.

The use of low dose intraoperative ketamine offers decreased postoperative pain and morphine consumption

Nonsteroidal anti-inflammatory drugs (NSAIDs) inhibit conversion of arachidonic acid to prostaglandin E2 in inflamed areas via cyclooxygenase (COX). It is suggested that the maximum daily dose of NSAIDs should be given/ordered because small doses of NSAIDs are not useful in acute pain relief [118]. When given in conjunction with opioids, NSAIDs reduced the postoperative opioid utilization and decreased unwanted opioid side effects [118].
NSAIDs should be used cautiously in those susceptible to its side effects including risk of renal injury, bleeding and peptic ulcers, asthma and bronchospasm. COX-2 selective inhibitors were developed to avoid the unwanted side effects of NSAIDs and may play a role as an adjunct in postoperative pain control.

4.3. Thoracic epidural

Thoracic epidural refers to analgesic technique of injecting medication into the epidural space, the potential space that surrounds the spinal cord. A segmental block results with coverage both above and below the injection site.

A single injection into the epidural space may be performed, or a catheter may be inserted for prolonged infusion. For post-thoracotomy pain relief, commonly a catheter is inserted via midline or paramedian technique in order to provide intermittent boluses as well as a continuous infusion for pain control. Infusions usually consist of a local anesthetic, an opioid, or a mixture of the two in order to optimize their synergistic effects [119] while reducing the individual doses and side effects [119, 120].

As the nerve roots leave the foramen and become peripheral nerves, they cross through the epidural space where they are bathed in the epidural solution.

Themechanismofactiondiffersbetweenlocalanestheticsandopioids.Localanestheticsblock sodium channels ultimately leading to blocked nerve conduction. The density of local anesthetic blockade is primarily dependent on the concentration of local anesthetic present, and dermatomal spread of blockade is dependent on the volume infused.

Also remember that the level of somatic block may be smaller than the sympathetic block because the somatic fibers are less sensitive [121]. Opioids bind to presynaptic and postsynaptic opioid receptors in the substantia gelatinosa, which inhibits the presynaptic release and postsynaptic response to neurotransmitters [121]. In a systemic review of randomized trials, Joshi et al. found that patients with thoracic epidural analgesia had a significantly lower pain score and needed less supplemental analgesia compared to systemic opioid analgesia.

Adverse effects may be from various aspects of epidural placement. Those associated with needle and catheter placement include back pain, inadvertent dural puncture, post-dural puncture headache, trauma to the spinal cord or nerves, and neuropathy (usually transient).

The dural puncture may lead to post-dural puncture headaches. The headache is usually characterized by severe fronto-occipital pain with head elevation that subsides, sometimes completely, upon return to the supine position [88].

The loss of CSF through the small puncture site may be enough to cause traction on the brain causing pain. Most patients' symptoms completely resolve after a few days to a week. Those that are not able or not willing to wait for spontaneous resolution may opt to undergo an epidural blood patch.

Neurologic injury may be the most feared complication of epidural analgesia. Nerve injury is usually transient and may occur from direct trauma to the nerves or spinal cord during needle insertion. A more devastating nerve injury can result from an epidural hematoma or abscess. Spinal hematoma occurs very rarely, approximately less than 1 in 150,000 [88].

Although rare, if it is not detected and treated promptly, it leads to irreversible paraplegia. The occurrence of hematoma has been on the rise, whether it is from increased coexistence of anticoagulation and regional anesthesia technique or from increased reporting [123]. Infection can occur from ineffective sterile preparation, contaminated drugs, an underlying infection, or bacteremia.

Any of these sources can cause an infection at the insertion site or lead to spread of infection from the skin along the indwelling catheter into the epidural space causing meningitis (if the dura was punctured) or abscess which could ultimately result in cord compression

Effects related to epidural injection of local anesthetic are usually dose related and include hypotension, motor block, systemic toxicity, and urinary retention. Epidural opioid administration may result in adverse effects that are similar to their parenteral administration.

These include pruritis, nausea, urinary retention, decreased arousability, ileus, and respiratory depression. Respiratory depression is the most concerning of the adverse effects and thus necessitates a monitored setting. After epidural injection, in the following 2-4 hours, early respiratory depression can occur which is likely due to the systemic absorption of the opioid[124]. Some opioids are more hydrophilic than others and have a tendency to remain in the CSF causing possible spread and delayed respiratory depression (usually occurs after 4 hours).

Relative contraindications to epidural include sepsis or bacteremia, infection at the insertion site, hypovolemia or shock, coagulopathy or thrombocytopenia, increased intracranial pressure (for risk of brain herniation if accidental dural puncture). One should use caution with patients who have underlying neurological diseases as not to confuse effects of the epidural versus pre-existing neurological deficits. The only absolute contraindication to epidural placement is patient refusal.

4.4. Thoracic paravertebral nerve block

TPVB involves injecting local anesthetic into the space adjacent to the thoracic vertebrae, which contains the spinal intercostal nerves. The boundaries of the space include the parietal pleura anterolaterally, the superior costotransverse ligament posteriorly, and medially by a portion of the vertebral body, intervertebral disc and intervertebral foramen [125]. The paravertebral space is continuous with the epidural space, intercostal space, and contralateral paravertebral space(by way of the prevertebral and epidural spaces).

intercostal space, and contralateral paravertebral space (by way of the prevertebral and epidural spaces). The caudal boundary of the space is at the origin of the psoas, while the cranial boundary is unknown. Cranially, radiographic dye has been noted after a thoracic paravertebral injection in the cervical area [126].

The intercostal nerves, dorsal rami, sympathetic chain and associated vessels lie within the fat of the paravertebral space [126]. A percutaneous technique is classically described whereby a needle is inserted into the space until a subtle loss of resistance is met followed by aspiration to ensure that the lung or pleura has not been breached before injecting small amounts of local anesthetic or insertion of a catheter [125].

The injection of local anesthetic can also be performed under direct visualization by the surgeon prior to the closure of the chest wall.

Injectionoflocalanestheticintotheparavertebralspa cecangivevaryingdegreesofanalgesia. The injection may remain localized to the area of injection producing a single level ipsilateral block, or it can spread to the above and below adjacent levels, as well as to the epidural space and contralateral paravertebral space. For example, Eason found that a single injection of 15mlof 0.375% bupivacaine spread over 4 spaces [125]. Similarly, 15ml of 0.5% bupivacaine injection led to a unilateral 5leveldermatome somatic block and8 level sympathetic block.

AdvantagesofTPVBaremany.TPVBiseasytolearnan dhasahighsuccessrate[126]. Successful placement of TPVB also can eliminate some unwanted effects of epidural analgesia such as spinal cord injury, spinal hematoma, excessive hypotension (owing to only a unilateral sympathetic blockade), and urinary retention [128]. Also, the nursing care required after TPVBis no different than normal post-surgical care [129]. A meta-analysis identified TPVB as having equivalent pain relief after thoracic surgery with less major side effects and decreased pulmonary complications to thatof epidural analgesia.

Adverse effects of TPVBinclude accidental pleural puncture, which could lead to a pneumothorax. The incidence of puncture and pneumothorax are 0.8% and 0.5% respectively, which is similar to other anesthetic procedures with pneumothorax risk [128]. Other adverse effects include relative hypotension, failed block, and vascular puncture.

ContraindicationstoTPVBaresimilartothoseofepidu ralplacementincludinginfectionat the insertion site, bacteremia, epyema. Another relative contraindication would be if the patient has had a previous thoracotomy because the ipsilateral paravertebral space may have been altered or obliterated as a result of surgery [124]. With respect to anticoagulation, the paravertebral space is less vascular than the epidural space, and paravertebral vessel puncture is less common.

4.5. Intercostal nerve block

The intercostal nerve provides sensory and motor innervation to chest wall and is found in the costal groove of each rib. Intercostal nerve blockade provides unilateral sensory and motor anesthesia to these areas. Local anesthetic is commonly injected 5 to 7 cm from the mid line over several sections owing to the great deal of overlap between the intercostal nerves.

There are different approaches to intercostal nerve blocks for thoracic procedures. The simplest is to inject local anesthetic around several intercostal nerves during thoracotomy when the chest wall is open. Cryotherapy, continuous infusion, or successive boluses of local anesthetic are also options.

Direct intercostal nerve block is most easily done by direct visualization during thoracotomy, but can also be done percutaneously.

Local is injected over multiple segments inferior to the rib with caution to avoid intravascular injection. Usually a small amount (2-5ml) of local is injected two to three spaces above and below the incision [131].

Cryoanalgesia interrupts nerve conduction for 1 to 3 months as a result of the freezing and subsequent damage of the myelin sheath [131] and is associated with long-term intercostal neuralgia [132].

Extrapleuralandinterpleuralinfusionoflocalanesthe ticarealsotechniquestoblock the intercostal nerves. Peeling back the pleura from the chest wall can create an extrapleural pocket, and a catheter can be introduced percutaneously into the space. After closure of the thoracotomy, an infusion of local anesthetic will fill the extrapleural space which leads to an intercostal block. Interpleural catheters can be inserted percutaneously to attain an intercostal nerve block, but one must keep in mind that a large volume of the anesthetic may be lost to the chest tubes. Interpleural anesthesia requires diffusion across the pleura and sub pleural space in order to attain an intercostal nerve blockade.

Single shot direct intercostal nerve block appears to have the same or superior pain control compared to epidural on the day of surgery, but after the effects of the local anesthesia have been exhausted, epidural anesthesia is superior to intercostal nerve block [131-133]

Detterbeckstatesthat extrapleural infusion of local anesthetic is more effective than systemic narcotics, and at least as good as thoracic epidural. Extrapleural intercostal nerve block provides a unilateral blockade, so the amount of urinary retention and hypotension are decreased, and there is not a need for special monitoring because the risk of respiratory depression is minimal [131]. Pain relief from intrapleural infusion is inconsistent

Systemic absorption of local anesthetic is notoriously high for intercostal nerve block due to the vascularity of the area of injection. There are no specific absolute contraindications to intercostal nerve blocks. They should be avoided for inpatients in whom high systemic levels of local anesthetics will not be well tolerated such as those with seizure disorders.

4.6. Elastomeric pumps

Wound infiltration with local anesthetic targets the peripheral level of pain and has been used widely in minor surgical procedures[134, 135]. The relatively short-term duration of the local infiltration limits the usefulness of one-time wound infiltration for more major thoracic surgery. An elastomeric pump connected to a multi-orifice catheter allows for continuous local anesthetic incisional infusion. Implementation of this technique is quite simple, with a minimal technical failure incidence [116].

A catheter is threaded in or near the insult and connected to a reservoir pump of local anesthetic by way of a flow-limiting valve. The surrounding tissues are then continuously bathed in the local anesthetic at 4ml/hr. By providing anesthesia at the site of insult there may be less need for systemic narcotics, and avoid many systemic narcotic effects including postoperative nausea and vomiting.

It is also believed that local anesthetic at the wound site can decrease the local inflammatory response which may in turn decrease pain and hyperalgesia[116]. Wheatley et al found that using an elastomeric pump is a safe and effective adjunct for post-thoracotomy pain relief.

Also, patients had lower pain scores and decreased narcotic need when compared to thoracic epidural analgesia alone [136]. Althoughlocalanesthetic toxicity is always a concern with infusions, the incidence of systemic toxicity is low [116]. Wound infiltration is safe and not associated with increased acute wound-related complications or long-term effects on wound healing.

4.7. Anticoagulation

Hemorrhagic complications from neuraxial blockade are of great concern.

Epidural analgesia is usually not initiated in patients who have a preexisting coagulopathy. The following are some consensus guidelines assembled by the American Society of Regional Anesthesia andPain Medicine[138]:

1.   Thrombolytic therapy

- Avoid thrombolytic for 10 days after neuraxial puncture,

- It is not clear how long to wait after thrombolytic therapy for the safe performance of neuraxial anesthesia.
- If neuraxial block is at or near the time of thrombolytic therapy neurologic checks should be none no less than every 2 hours,

- There is no recommendation for the removal of neuraxial catheters in unexpected thrombolytic therapy

2.   Subcutaneous unfractionated heparin

- Review of other medications that may affect clotting is advised

- There is little risk of spinal hematoma
- Placementoftheblockpriortotherapymaybedesirablealthoughincreasedriskisnot demonstrated in the presence of subcutaneous heparin

- In twice-daily doses–epidurals may be placed before the next scheduled dose, the catheter can coexist with the regimen, and preferably the catheter can be removed one hour prior to next dose

- Thrice daily doses or more than 10,000units unfractionated heparin–there is no data published, but it is advised not to maintain an epidural catheter with this regimen

- If the patient has received more than four days of heparin, a platelet count should be obtained prior to block or removal of the catheter in the instance of heparin-induced thrombocytopenia.

- After needle placement, wait one hour to administer heparin.

- Wait 2-4hours after heparin to remove catheters, resume therapy one hour after removal of catheter

- Bloody placement may increase the risk of hematoma, but the case does not necessarily need to be cancelled.

3. Low-Molecular Weight Heparin

- A bloody placement does not mandate cancellation of the case, however, LMWH should be delayed for 24 hours

- Epidural placement should happen 10-12 hours after last dose

- If the patient is on higher dose LMWH, one should wait 24 hours to place epidural • Do not place epidural at 2 hours after dose – peak anticoagulation activity

- Twice daily doses should not be initiated with an indwelling catheter and must be removed before the first dose

- Once-daily dosing – may start 6-8 hours postoperatively, the catheter can be maintained, removal after 10-12 hours of the last dose

4. Oral Anticoagulants – Warfarin

- INR should be normalized prior to the neuraxial technique

- If initial dose of warfarin is given more than 24 hours prior to surgery, INR should be checked prior to neuraxial block

- If low-dose warfarin therapy is ongoing during epidural anesthesia, neurological evaluations and daily INR checks are advised

- Catheters should be removed when INR is less than 1.5, and neurological assessment should be continuedfor24 hours

- If 1.5< INR< 3, catheters should be cautiously removed

- If the INR is more than3, the dose of warfarin should be held/reduced

5. Antiplatelet Medications

- NSAIDs have no specific concerns or added risk with epidural with or without catheter placement unless concurrent medications affecting clotting

- The risk of bleeding with clopidogrel, ticlopidine, and GP IIB/IIIA inhibitors is not known.

- 7 and 14 days should elapse between discontinuation of ticlopidine and clopidogre, respectively, and placement of neuraxial block

- Platelet function normalization must occur before placement of neuraxial block if discontinued for only 5-7days

- Epidural catheters should not be maintained while on GP IIB/IIIA inhibitor therapy

6. Herbals

- They do not create risk that impedes with neuraxial block
- Garlic inhibits platelet aggregation, increases fibrinolysis
- Ginko inhibits platelet-activating factor
- Ginseng has the potential to inhibit coagulation7.   Thrombin inhibitors
- Monitored by a PTTT

- Anticoagulation effect present for 1-3hours
- There are no pharmacologic reversal
- Neuraxial techniques are best avoided

8. Fondaparinux

- Factor Xa inhibitor

- Unknown risk of spinal hematoma

5. Conclusion

The challenges of thoracic anesthesia are unique among all anesthetic subspecialties. Its practitioners must be well-versed in a wide range of anesthetic management principles, from advanced airway techniques to ventilations strategies and pain management. The two subspecialties of thoracic surgery and thoracic anesthesia continue to co-evolve to improve patient safety and surgical outcomes

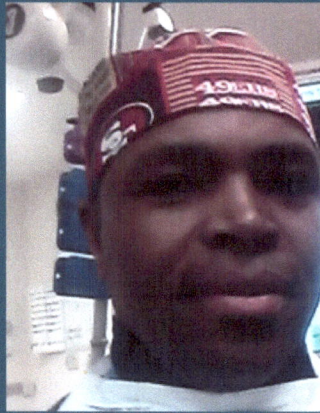

Author: Tonypang

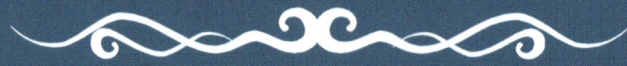

www.ingramcontent.com/pod-product-compliance
Lightning Source LLC
Chambersburg PA
CBHW061139030426
42335CB00002B/46